Citizen's Guide
to Health Care Reform

Understanding the Affordable Care Act

D1456504

Robert L. McCan, Ph.D.

Quantity discounts are available for educational purposes, bulk sales, promotions, premiums, fundraising, and group study. Special editions or bound excerpts of the book may be created for specific groups or purposes in collaboration with the author.

Contact the author, Robert L. McCan, at 513 West Broad Street, Suite 517, Falls Church, Virginia 22046 or through his website: www.BobMcCan.com.

First 2012 Election Edition published April 2012.

ISBN-13: 978-1475010350

ISBN-10: 1475010354

LCCN: 2012905183

Printed by CreateSpace, Charleston, South Carolina.

Published by Robert L. McCan, Ph.D., Falls Church, Virginia.

TABLE OF CONTENTS

4 COST CONTROL 103

PROLOGUE: A MEDICARE MEMOIR
Context for the Affordable Care Act

I was reared in a Missouri town of 1,200 and emerged into adulthood at the beginning of World War II. I often heard the story of my grandfather, a farmer, who died at age 45, ten years before I was born. The cause of death was an appendix rupture. There was only one doctor for a large rural population, but he had minimal medical training and no way to perform surgery. The closest hospital was 80 miles away in St. Louis at a time when automobiles were just making their debut. My grandfather died before he could be put on a train to the city, leaving a distraught widow and four children, my mother being the youngest. Decades later, I could still see the pain in my grandmother's face when she remembered the day her husband died. I knew a routine operation probably would have saved his life. I believed in universal coverage before I had any inkling of public policy issues.

Doctors were as scarce as hen's teeth in our town when I was growing up; indeed, the first accredited doctor arrived during my senior year of high school. The town celebrated when the young physician, Charles Brenner, opened a practice on the lower level of his house. Personally, I had never been in a doctor's office until after I graduated from high school. It was Dr. Brenner who gave me a pre-induction exam when I applied to join the U.S. Navy at age 19.

After college and the war I attended Yale University Divinity School for three years on the G.I. Bill and was then ordained as a Baptist minister. I spent the next five years at the First Baptist Church in Marshall, Missouri, a county seat town of 10,000 and the home of Missouri Valley College. My ministry extended to a significant group of local college students, one of whom was Blue Carstenson, who became a friend and colleague years later. As a college student he was a budding activist. Social justice was his religion. I supported his activism: we decided to undertake a project to build public housing for the African American poor of our town. He enlisted the professor of his sociology class and the entire class embarked on a survey of substandard housing. I gave a sermon revealing the abysmal survey findings and then spoke on the topic to the student body at a college assembly. We soon learned that we needed enabling legislation from the state before we could begin a low income housing project. We stirred the waters, but in the end Blue graduated and I moved away before any houses were built.

Five years to the day after arriving in Marshall I resigned and moved with my wife and daughters, ages 5 and 4, to Edinburgh, Scotland, where I enrolled in a doctoral program in theology and ethics. While we were living in Edinburgh, our older daughter needed her tonsils removed and we were introduced to the British medical system. We were impressed. Suzy had a competent general practice doctor, a good surgeon and adequate hospital care. She got appropriate medications to take home, and a visiting nurse came to see her regularly until she recovered fully. The total cost to us as visitors: zero.

I made many inquiries about the National Health System, which in 1953 had been in existence only five years. In general, people had minor gripes, but they were thrilled to have peace of mind and medical security. Doctors were less uniformly pleased, but most had settled into the system and accepted the value of universal coverage. The salary scale gave the doctors an upper middle class life style. Specialists who had been making much more money were the most dissatisfied.

I became a believer after my experience in Edinburgh. From that time forward a part of my Christian commitment to a public policy ethic was the right of every person to basic health care.

Fast forward to 1955: I was the minister of the First Baptist Church in Clarksville, Tennessee and a member of the Christian Life Commission for Southern Baptists, offering leadership on difficult social and political issues. In the spring of 1956, I attended the Southern Baptist Convention in Chicago and learned that, as our meeting ended, the Democratic National Committee would be convening there. It was billed as a major event, with most Democratic Senators and Representatives attending. They would make plans for the national election in the fall. I decided to stay and see how much I could attend.

The first meeting was an expensive luncheon at the Blackstone Hotel and the topic was whether to make national health insurance a primary plank in the platform. I slipped into the large banquet hall as dessert was being served and stayed until the session ended at 4:00 p.m. At least a hundred persons spoke. The sentiment was ten to one in favor of a strong campaign for national health insurance. Most of those who opposed were doctors or persons otherwise tied to the medical profession. I remember one young U.S. Representative who spoke with unusual passion. I failed to get his name and after the speech I turned to the person next to me to ask who he was. He replied, "That is the new Congressman from Minnesota, Hubert Humphrey."

A huge rally was held on Saturday night at Wrigley Field, attended by 40,000 enthusiastic Democrats. The primary speakers were former President Harry Truman and Adlai Stevenson, Governor of Illinois. Both rang the bells in support of health care for all. I felt assured that with all of the excitement and urgency, the national insurance program would surely be enacted. But alas, Eisenhower won a second term. He was not a major reformer, so the vision had to wait for another day.

My challenging and busy ministry passed quickly and in 1960 I moved to the First Baptist Church of Danville, Virginia. My vision was for a ministry that balanced social justice and personal faith set in a loving community. John Kennedy was President. I followed carefully, though at a distance, the new debate over Medicare. I knew that Kennedy had read the political tea leaves and discerned that a national health bill could not pass, so he had narrowed the focus and proposed national health insurance for seniors only. The controversy came close to home, as there were 27 medical doctors in my congregation, 25 of them strongly opposed to Medicare. The medical community across the country was leading the opposition to Medicare, especially in the South. I found it hard to fathom their heated condemnation of the British health care system, including their insistence that the British people hated it.

Then one day in 1962 the phone rang in my office and at the other end of the line was Blue Carstenson. We had lost contact after the summer of 1953. I remembered only that he had enrolled in the University of Michigan and planned to work for a doctorate in Adult Education with the expectation of becoming a YMCA executive. Blue explained that he was Executive Director of the National Council of Senior Citizens (NCSC) in Washington, D.C. and he had previously served at the sub-cabinet level as Director of Adult Education for the United States. He explained that President Kennedy had asked him to lead the senior organization and make it into an advocacy organization for Medicare. The reason for his call was to ask if I would speak in support of Medicare at a college-wide assembly. He said a faculty committee at Hampden-Sydney College had gotten a doctor from the American Medical Association to speak to the faculty and students on the Medicare issue. The speaker had been totally against Medicare. The faculty committee in charge of arranging assemblies had called Blue to ask if he would come to present the case for Medicare. Unfortunately, Blue was too busy to go. Blue explained to me that he had followed my career from afar and knew that I was in Danville, Virginia. He asked me to speak in his place.

I went to the college and presented the case for Medicare. Unbeknownst to me at the time, the Danville medical society had hired someone to go to Farmville and tape my address. That very night the doctors met to listen to the tape of my speech favoring Medicare. Stormy weather followed, primarily from the 25 medical doctors in my congregation who opposed Medicare, but the pilings were driven deep enough under my professional house that I endured the storm.

After three years in Danville I found myself swirling in another storm that I could not weather. We were in the middle of the racial upheaval of the 1960s. I had organized the Danville Council on Human Relations to build bridges for racial fellowship and understanding. Martin Luther King, Jr. came to Danville. There were marches and sit-ins. 230 demonstrators ended up in jail. The mainline ministers in the downtown churches stood unified in support of the goals of Martin Luther King, Jr. Of the 15 churches, including mine, 14 fired their ministers within a month.

It was time for me to make an assessment. I concluded, with deep regret, that Southern Baptists were moving rapidly toward a fundamentalist takeover where I would not be welcome. Further, in those days it was hard to find employment at another church when one had lost a position because of a stand on race. I also questioned whether my call any longer was to a congregation when, it seemed, so many members opposed a ministry of peace and social justice. I decided to leave the pastoral ministry and set my sights on forming an international college, where young people could learn to live together in the global village of tomorrow.

To prepare for this new endeavor, I went back to school at Harvard University as a Visiting Scholar with faculty status. I wanted to learn how to become a good college president while developing a philosophy of education for the college of the future.

During my second year at Harvard I accepted a one-year faculty appointment at Boston University School of Education. Later, I was offered a permanent faculty position there. During this time I was further developing my vision of the college, with the help of a hundred graduate students. We decided the college should be located in the Washington, D.C. area.[1]

The phone rang one evening at my residence and to my great surprise Dr. J. Earl Williams was on the line. He was a university professor of labor economics who five years earlier had been an active member of my congregation in Clarksville, Tennessee. He had just accepted the invitation of Sargent Shriver to direct Employment Programs in the new U.S. Office of Economic Opportunity. Earl invited me to be the Associate Director and I gladly accepted.

Soon after arriving in the nation's capital I contacted Blue Carstenson and we began a renewed friendship and a professional working relationship. He told me his story. While a student at the University of Michigan he had volunteered to work in the second Presidential campaign of Adlai Stevenson at his headquarters in Chicago. He was put in charge of logistics, assigning office spaces and secretarial help to high level volunteers. A young man came in one day asking to help for the remainder of the campaign. He introduced himself to Blue as Jack Kennedy, a U.S. Representative from Massachusetts. They worked together and became friends.

Four years later Jack Kennedy became the Democratic candidate for president. Blue had just finished his doctorate in adult education. Kennedy asked Blue to serve as an advance man for his campaign, and later he invited him to join his personal campaign staff. After he won the election Kennedy appointed Blue as Director of Adult Education for the nation. A few months later, Blue said he got a call from the President's secretary asking him to come by the Oval Office. The President explained how much he wanted to enact universal national health insurance legislation. Since that seemed politically impossible at the time, he had decided to pull out all the stops to pass Medicare, a national health insurance program for seniors. The President said he had been around long enough to know that even this limited plan would not pass the Congress unless a very strong constituency of older people could be mobilized to lobby for it. He asked Blue to leave Adult Education and assume leadership of the National Council of Senior Citizens. He told Blue how he appreciated his relentless drive to get him elected. He expected Blue to display that same singular focus to pass Medicare.

Blue told me he took the job with two goals in mind: first, build the NCSC base from 25,000 to a million if necessary, and second, lobby until Medicare became law.

When President Kennedy was killed in Dallas, Texas, President Johnson asked Blue to continue his efforts and even redouble them in order to make Medicare a monument to Kennedy. Johnson also expanded the Peace Corps and started the War on Poverty with the support of Congress, again billed as tributes to Kennedy.

The process of explaining the value of Medicare to members of Congress and convincing them to pass a law providing universal health care for seniors was long and difficult. The country had never had any type of national health insurance before. Blue's efforts were creative and convincing. One of his most successful events happened when he led 30,000 senior citizens to Philadelphia to the 1964 Democratic National Convention, where LBJ was nominated for a full term. They marched. They lobbied. They got publicity across the country and made a strong impression on the convention floor.

What really changed the landscape was the resounding victory of LBJ in November 1964 and the historic change in the composition of the House and Senate. Most of the new Democratic members had campaigned on a "Fair Deal" platform in the "Great Society" with Medicare as a major plank. LBJ's victory came the year before I moved to Washington.

We return to 1965 when I accepted Dr. J. Earl Williams' offer to be the Associate Director for Employment Programs at the U.S. Office of Economic Opportunity. That year I was extremely busy working on employment programs for poor persons.

Unbelievably, at that time there were no programs in the War on Poverty that focused on the elderly. Blue at the National Council of Senior Citizens and others at the National Council on Aging, the national professional organization, were distressed by this failure to include the elderly. Once again, older persons were ignored and bypassed. Sargent Shriver's rationale was to focus on programs for the young, where there seemed to be more bang for the buck. Blue talked with me about what could be done to include older persons. One obvious route was to enlist support from the Senate Select Committee on Aging.

Senators got on board, none more than Ted Kennedy, Sargent Shriver's brother-in-law. They pushed Shriver to create a department with programs for the elderly. In the end, he compromised. Instead of a full-blown department, he established an office. Instead of a separate structure, he placed it in the Employment Division. Sargent Shriver appointed me, with Earl Williams' recommendation, as the first Acting Director of Older Persons Programs in the U.S. Office of Economic Opportunity.

Now Blue and I worked more closely together. When Congress was in session, Blue and I would go to the Capitol in the evening. We would pace the halls outside the legislative chambers, walking in step with any Congress-person who was alone. All Congress members knew him by this time. He had actively campaigned in the 1964 election season for those who favored Medicare and had helped to defeat many who opposed it. The momentum for his lobby was growing. A Gallup Poll at the time revealed that 67% of the people in the country favored Medicare, although a majority did not understand exactly what was in the bill.

Blue also contributed ideas to my office. He suggested employment programs for seniors, one of which is still in operation some 45 years later. Green Thumb was his idea. We began Green Thumb employment programs in 18 states, hiring older farmers to work in highway beautification. They worked 20 hours a week at minimum wage which more than doubled their incomes, since many farmers did not participate in Social Security. They did what they did best—make things grow—and they garnered a lot of recognition and appreciation. It was a favorite program of Lady Bird Johnson. When I invited a representative of each state program to Washington for feedback on the projects, Lady Bird invited the 18 men, ages 68 to 90, and me to the White House for a tour and for tea with her in the library.

To get a clear picture of how Medicare finally passed through Congress, we must understand the work of Wilbur D. Mills, (D. Ark.), Chairman of the House Ways and Means Committee and arguably the most powerful man in Congress at the time. He was a conservative southern Representative and instinctively opposed Medicare, but he was also a consummate politician who wanted to lead the march and not fall behind the troops. In an effort to preempt Medicare he had sponsored, along with Senator Robert Kerr, (D. Okla.) the Kerr-Mills bill, passed in 1960 and known as Medical Assistance for the Aging (MAA), which provided some medical aid to the elderly poor. However, only 28 states decided to participate, and many of these kept budgets for the program too low to meet needs.

Mills continued to oppose the Medicare legislation until the 1964 election, when he saw the writing on the wall. He was determined to lead whatever bill became law. As a conservative, he at first proposed only what is now Part A, hospital insurance, as the Medicare Bill. But the more liberal Democrats and Medicare supporters around the country demanded more. They discussed coverage of doctors' bills and other medical expenses for the older person who was not in the hospital. As a compromise, Part B was added, but the recipient had to request it and share in paying the cost.

The House Ways and Means Committee marked up the bill behind closed doors in off-the-record sessions with a two-thirds margin of Democrats. Remarkably, no member of the American Medical Association was invited to testify. Representative Durwood Hall (R. Mo.), a physician, commented on the House floor, "at no time during the week this bill was drafted were the nation's doctors asked to contribute to the deliberations." He called it "the most brazen act of omission ever committed on a piece of legislation."[2] Lyndon Johnson worked the phones and twisted arms in the days leading up to the vote. The House passed the Medicare Bill 313 to 115 on April 8, 1965. The Senate voted, after the Conference with the House to reconcile the Bills, on July 29, 1965. The vote was 70 to 24 in favor, and President Johnson signed the bill into law the next day, July 30, 1965.

Late in the afternoon of July 29, I got a telephone call from Blue inviting me to come that evening to the Hilton Hotel at 16th and K Streets for a celebration. First, he penned a newsletter to the million members of NCSC, sharing the good news. It was a time to rejoice and reflect on the long journey. Members of Congress heaped praise on those who had taken the political heat. None spoke with greater joy or eloquence than Hubert Humphrey, and Blue was cheered for his relentless pursuit of the prize.

President Johnson decided to go to Independence, Missouri so he could sign the Medicare bill into law in the presence of Harry Truman, the then old warrior-champion of universal health care. He invited Blue, some staff directors, and leading Members of Congress to accompany him on Air Force One. When he signed the Medicare Act into law, the first pen went to Harry Truman and the second pen went to Blue Carstenson.

The final legislation resulted in the creation of Medicare Parts A and B. Upon enactment, everyone age 65 and older was automatically enrolled in Part A, the hospital insurance, but seniors needed to choose Part B to cover doctor bills, x-rays and a host of other medical expenses. Seniors who chose Part B paid a modest amount monthly from their Social Security checks. The cost was (and is) extremely small compared to the benefits. The new law provided a specific time frame for initial enrollment into Part B.

Blue and I conferred over how we might construct an older persons' employment program in OEO that would inform older poor persons about the benefits of Part B. We feared that most of them would not understand the "legalese" in the brochures sent out by the Social Security administration and would fail to enroll. I wrote a proposal to Sargent Shriver suggesting that we employ older poor persons to go door to door in targeted areas and tell the story, so seniors would enroll. The legal team at OEO turned down my audacious idea. The Social Security Administration blanched at the thought of having older uneducated persons explaining the new Medicare law. They foresaw multiple lawsuits. The boss threw the proposal in the waste basket. It was too dangerous.

The Senate Select Committee on Aging began to place calls to Sargent Shriver, the most irate from Ted Kennedy, demanding that the proposal be funded. The National Council on Aging was on board and Blue enlisted other Congressional allies. Finally, Mr. Shriver got the proposal out of the waste basket and signed it. Unfortunately, we had a short window of time before the enrollment deadline. My assistant, Jack Ossofsky (who from 1971 to 1988 led the National Council on Aging), and I sent a notice to Community Action Agency Directors across the nation asking them to come to a meeting at one of the seven government regional centers. We would meet them there, explain the program and show them how to apply for a grant. I went to four cities in four days and Jack went to three. We had designed an abbreviated two-page application form, which, by miracle, we got approved within days. I wrote a report for the Director when the project ended. 30,000 older poor persons had visited three million seniors and explained to them the benefits of Medicare, Part B. There was never a hint of a lawsuit.

A Postscript

When my life was focused on passing Medicare, however small my part, I was not thinking of my own parents any more than many millions of other older persons in America, most without health insurance. It never occurred to me that the blessings of the new law would impact me personally. Some years later, however, my father, age 73, was given an experimental drug for gout. The drug, later withdrawn from the market because of unacceptable side effects, destroyed his body's ability to make white blood cells. He needed blood transfusions to live. He had neither the mind-set nor the financial resources to sue the drug company to cover the cost. I was deeply grateful that he had Medicare, allowing his life to be extended for another three years.

I rejoiced again decades later when the Patient Protection and Affordable Care Act passed Congress and President Obama signed it into law in March of 2010. I was dismayed, however, by people's lack of knowledge of what the law contained. It seemed that opponents had just one purpose—to confuse the public and distort the terms of the law. Even supposedly knowledgeable media pundits showed a remarkable ignorance of what was in the law. So, I took up the project of studying the legislation, the issues, and the political forces surrounding it. I offer what I hope is a factual account of the content of the new law, combined with my deeply held opinions and perspectives. We have another rare opportunity to move toward universal coverage and to improve health care for most Americans!

Chapter 1

THE AFFORDABLE CARE ACT:

AN OVERVIEW

The United States is the only wealthy, industrialized
nation that does not have a universal health care system.
 –Institute of Medicine, National Academy of Sciences

How do we create a health care system that covers everyone with higher quality care at a lower cost?

In March 2010 Congress passed and President
Obama signed into law the Patient Protection and
Affordable Care Act (ACA). The 1,000+ page law,[3] with its
legal language and mind-numbing detail, addresses three
simple purposes. Woven through its pages like three
golden threads, are answers to these three questions:

1. Inclusion: How do we include every citizen? Can
   we all go to the doctor, get good hospital care, use
   appropriate diagnostic equipment, and receive the
   most effective treatments?
2. Quality: How can we improve the quality of health
   services for every American, from the poorest to the
   richest? How can we improve the nation's health?
3. Cost: How can we lower the cost, or at least
   dramatically curb the rate at which health costs are
   climbing? Can we get costs under control?

It would be much easier if we could answer one or even two of these questions and omit the third. We could readily increase quality of care if we didn't need to worry about cost. Or, we could more easily control cost if we didn't need to bring another 32 million citizens into the system, more than half of whom cannot afford the full cost of insurance. However, as we shall see, the law represents a commitment to addressing all three of these challenging issues.

The Law's Potential Impact

This is one of the most comprehensive, far-reaching laws of the last hundred years. It is as far-reaching for the entire population as Social Security and Medicare have been for the elderly. Yet, the law's impact is not immediately apparent. It will be phased in gradually over many years, with January 1, 2014 as a pivotal date. Despite its critical importance, this is a modest law. It provides a weaker system of health care than that found in any other industrialized nation. Most Democrats wanted a "single-payer" plan. They sought to eliminate the inefficiencies and costly expenditures inherent in for-profit plans and profit centers.

The Affordable Care Act, in fact, was the Republican plan during the years when Democrats pushed for more extensive reform. It is similar to the most comprehensive plan enacted into law by a state — Massachusetts. Republican Governor Mitt Romney shepherded that bill through the Massachusetts legislature in 1996 and signed it into law as a cardinal Republican achievement. He presented it as an exercise in common sense and personal responsibility. That was before candidate Obama decided to adopt this conservative approach. He wanted to win bipartisan support and avoid a big battle with the pharmaceutical companies, private insurers, doctors and the hospital systems—entrenched interests that had torpedoed earlier attempts to enact health care reform. Republicans had previously supported this basic approach, if not all of the details, as a way to deal with our out-of-control system—until the President and his staff invited Governor Romney's team of advisors to come to White House on numerous occasions and help write the outline of a plan that Democrats accepted only very reluctantly.

Richard Nixon supported this concept in the 1970s, working with Senator Edward Kennedy. In a special message to Congress[4] on February 6, 1974, President Nixon presented his plan, insisting that it include seven points:

1. Every American would be covered.
2. Each American would pay only as much as the person could afford.
3. The new system would retain and build on the existing system of private health insurance.
4. Public funds would be used only where needed.'
5. The plan would retain freedom of choice for doctors and patients.
6. The plan would look at the system as a whole and make it more efficient.
7. All parties would have a direct stake in making the system work.

President Nixon's plan was quite similar to the Affordable Care Act. George H.W. Bush also endorsed the basic concept in the 1980s. Robert Dole added his support in 1994 when it was the standard Republican position. The "mandate," now a major bone of contention for Republicans, had been endorsed in recent years by such leading Republicans as John McCain, Charles Grassley, Oren Hatch, Lindsey Graham and Scott Brown. Indeed, several of these Republican senators actually co-sponsored legislation that included a mandate, while the conservative Heritage Foundation provided policy research that supported it. Again, all of that support came before President Obama adopted the approach. Once the Democrats accepted it, the Republicans transfigured the plan into an evil beyond redemption.

Building on the Existing System

The new law builds on our existing system, which includes both private and public components. It embraces the existence of 1,300 private insurance companies, while requiring all of them to meet certain minimum standards. As of 2011, 45% of people got insurance through private health plans sponsored by their employers. Authors of the bill assume that this percentage will hold firm or increase over time, as has happened in Massachusetts. This, however, would be a reversal of the trend downward, as each year the percentage getting insurance from employers has declined due to the rapidly rising cost. The self-employed can get insurance in the current system, but their rates are higher because they are not in large pools. The new law congregates these individuals into large groups, enabling them to be covered at a lower cost.

Active military personnel will continue to have their own government-run health system known as the

Military Health Service, and eligible veterans will still have access to government-run Veterans' Health Administration (VHA) hospitals and clinics. TRICARE is a program that funds private insurance for military dependents. The nation has 23 million veterans and 8.3 million of them, about the population of Virginia, receive care through the VHA system. The VHA employs 200,000 administrators, doctors, nurses and other health professionals. It operates 152 hospitals and 784 outpatient clinics with an annual budget of $50 billion.

Community Health Centers (CHC) are a little-known component of our health care system, established about 40 years ago to provide primary care in underserved areas, mostly rural. They are administered through the Health Resources and Services Administration of HHS, with a budget of $7.5 billion in 2010. There were about 1,100 CHCs serving 20 million people when the Affordable Care Act was passed in 2010.

Medicare is the largest government health-related program, with 47.5 million beneficiaries and expenditures of $523 billion in 2010. It is an insurance program; actual medical services are provided in the free-enterprise marketplace. Citizens age 65 and older have been assured since Medicare passed in 1965 that they need never fear for lack of basic medical care. While the goal of universal coverage has been achieved for the Medicare age group, a major focus of the ACA is controlling the rapidly escalating costs of the program while improving quality and health outcomes. Medicare is revised and incorporated into the new law.

Another piece of our health care pie is the Children's Health Insurance Program (CHIP). Many low-income children are overlooked by Medicaid, the primary low-income government health care program. Others with parents somewhat above the poverty line still can't get proper medical care. Their parents cannot afford to spend scarce funds for their medical checkups, shots, dental care or for major accidents or illnesses. Senators Ted Kennedy (D. Mass.) and Orrin Hatch (R. Utah) first sponsored the bi-partisan CHIP legislation in 1997. In FY2009, approximately 7.7 million children were enrolled in CHIP. Federal expenditures were $7.5 billion, with an additional $3.1 billion contributed by the states. CHIP has been upgraded and incorporated into the new law as another way to increase coverage.

Finally, there is Medicaid, the second largest health-related program. Total expenditures in FY2009 were $378.6 billion, including both federal and state government contributions. Most citizens served by this program are below the poverty line. They simply do not make enough money to pay for insurance or the expensive medical care offered in today's marketplace.

When we add up these parts of the existing system (private insurance provided mostly through employers and public programs that include the U.S. military, CHCs, Medicare, CHIP, and Medicaid), we cover some 250 million Americans. Unfortunately, 50 million are still left without insurance. How do we bring the uninsured under the umbrella of protection? Some of these 50 million include the wealthy few who choose to self-insure. Others are temporarily unemployed or in the process of changing jobs and will get insurance as soon as they are settled.

These two categories account for 15 to 18 million persons who will presumably have access to medical care through existing channels. This leaves some 32 million in the other categories of the uninsured.

Also among the uninsured are the young and healthy and others who could afford health insurance but assume no illness will befall them and simply choose not to pay for coverage. These people are willing to take a chance, save money and hope to get by without insurance protection. However, the people who feel they are above the fray are the minority. The majority of this uninsured one-sixth of the population is simply financially unable to afford insurance.

The new law requires the uninsured to get coverage like everyone else. Those who can afford a minimum level policy must enroll in a private plan, using an online insurance "exchange" set up by their state. This is the "coverage mandate" that has stirred more controversy than any other feature of the law. One purpose for a coverage mandate is to spread the risk more evenly across a broader base of the population. The mandate makes it possible for the insurance companies to fulfill the other more popular provisions of the new law such as covering people with pre-existing conditions and not dropping people from coverage after they get an expensive illness. Even those who are healthy now will benefit from the encouragement to get regular checkups, appropriate screenings, and other services focused on prevention that presumably prevent higher costs in the future. This may seem unfair and expensive to the young and healthy, but in reality, it serves both them and the larger society. It also mitigates emergency room use, the most expensive way to receive care. In fact, many ER visits are for colds and common ailments and could be more effectively treated by primary care physicians. **The success of the Affordable Care Act depends on having every citizen enrolled in some sort of insurance, whether public or private.**

How do we include that segment of the population that can afford some payment but not the full cost of insurance? The Affordable Care Act raises the minimum eligibility for Medicaid from 100% to 133% of the poverty line, while reducing states' ability to vary eligibility standards. People with incomes above 400% of the federal poverty line will be required to purchase at least a minimum policy at their own expense. Those who make between 133% and 400% of the federal poverty line will pay on an established sliding scale, with a federal subsidy for the portion they can't afford.

Of the newly insured, the split between Medicaid and subsidized private insurance is expected to be about 50-50. Of the 32 million uninsured persons in this pool, the law is expected by 2019 to cover about 16 million under Medicaid and the other 16 million in exchanges with private insurance, subsidized by the federal government.

There it is. That is the plan for universal coverage with many varieties of flowers growing side by side in a health care garden. This is health care "lite," when compared to proposals by Presidents Truman, Kennedy, Johnson, Nixon and Clinton.

Regulating the Insurance Companies

The law seeks to lower costs, in part by regulating insurance providers. Any insurance company that wishes to participate in the exchanges to be established state by state must meet minimum requirements. It must be registered in that state, as it is now. Of course, it must continue to have financial resources sufficient to assure payment of claims. Adoption of standardized or compatible electronic billing and records is a new requirement. This should substantially reduce the overhead costs and inefficiencies incurred by providers who maintain large clerical staffs to handle billings and a host of differing forms and paperwork imposed by each company. An ACA requirement is that the records of each company must be compatible with the computerized forms used by all other providers. The details of each plan offered in a given state must be posted online in a consistent format, along with the exact cost to a consumer. Their profit and loss and a record of claims paid and claims denied must also be transparent, reported regularly, and presented in a standardized form for government audit.

Each company must demonstrate that it operates efficiently and pays out in medical services 80% to 85% of every dollar received from customers, including the government. There is room for profit and for reasonable executive salaries, but no tax deductions are allowed on salaries and incentives above $500,000 annually for executives. Any insurance company that collects more than the 15% to 20% allowed for overhead and profit must refund the excess to enrollees the next year. The law further establishes an appeal process in each state exchange, so that a person who believes he or she is not being treated fairly according to the terms of the law can appeal to an independent board.

Organizing into Exchanges

Insurance providers will sell their various health plans in an online marketplace called an insurance exchange. Each state will have one exchange whose purpose is to create competition and variety, so enrollees have clear choices and lowest costs. Each insurance company will offer four plans, with coverage of cost from 90% down to 60%. Large companies have traditionally self-financed their own health plans and contracted directly with doctors, hospitals and other providers for services to their employees. By controlling their system they have offered the most benefits at the lowest cost. These companies are not required to use the exchanges, and most will probably choose to keep their current programs for health care. Nonetheless, all insurance plans are now required to meet the standards of the exchanges. Many of the cost saving measures in all plans are adopted from the pioneering work of large corporations.

A second category, small employers, will use the exchange to participate in a large pool so they can obtain the same low rates as large companies. Because small companies often operate at lower profits, the government will pay a part of the premium cost as a way to protect small business.

The third type of policy in the exchange covers the self-employed. Individual policies, traditionally the most expensive, will now garner the same kind of savings as others in the exchanges. This pool will also include employees whose companies, large or small, do not provide insurance.

Finally, there are government-assisted citizens between 133% and 400% of the poverty line whose premiums will be partially subsidized. By grouping these people into the large pool, the new system reduces their premium costs. Medicare and Medicaid in each state negotiate rates separately, using federal guidelines.

Each state by law must have a non-profit insurance cooperative as one of the insurance providers. The Act calls them Consumer-Owned and Oriented Plans (CO-OP). $6 billion in federal funds was authorized to create and support these plans that are expected to operate primarily in individual and small-group markets. Proponents say these organizations can serve members better because they focus on service rather than profits. CO-OPs are expected to provide good coverage, reduced rates; they will compete with private insurers. These cooperatives will be self-governed by elected boards of their members. They will determine premiums, benefits, deductibles, and co-pays. Health insurance cooperatives will be exempt from federal taxes. The Department of Health and Human Services (HHS) is working on guidelines; grants and loans are expected to be awarded by July 1, 2013. Insurance industry insiders are skeptical of the ability of CO-OPs to deal with the tangles of finance, legal responsibility and medical complexity. Ideally, from the perspective of those who wrote the law, they will be able to operate efficiently and challenge the costs of private plans.

Some national insurance companies may decide to enter every state exchange. They must declare this intention, win federal approval and meet each state's standards. The first year, 2014, they must be approved in 60% of states, the next year in 70%, and so on until the company operates in every state by 2017. A half dozen or more insurance companies are expected to compete in each large state exchange. In areas of the country with small state populations, only one or two companies might choose to offer policies. Hence, some states may join with neighboring states to form a multi-state exchange that will assure the necessary number of companies for competition to become effective.

Starting in 2014 large employers must pay up to $3,000 as an annual assessment for employees who are denied in-house coverage. Companies can, if they prefer, provide their employees with vouchers for a specific annual amount for health insurance, rather than negotiate directly with a single provider or provide their own internal health plan, as is done now. The employees, in turn, take their vouchers to the exchange, choose both the insurance company and the specific policy they want and use the vouchers to credit their costs. This gives employees a level of choice usually lacking now.

In the beginning the exchange will serve primarily the small business market, the self-employed, and the retired who are not old enough for Medicare. It will also serve that population eligible for subsidies. The first year of operation will be 2014 when eight million persons are expected to use the exchanges. The framers of the Act estimate that 24 million will use them by 2018 and the number will continue to grow as companies and individuals see the many advantages. Prices will vary, depending on cost of living in a specific location, plan level chosen, and age, as is true today.

The Consumer of Health Services

From your perspective as a health care consumer, you will go online to your state department of health or other designated server to find an appropriate policy. The website has a basic information form that asks about your income, medical needs and place of employment. Based on that information, it then displays multiple plans that fit your circumstance. If you qualify for Medicaid, Medicare, or a private insurance subsidy, the system identifies that for you. You then review the various policies offered by several insurance companies in your state, read online comments by other customers, and compare the costs and provisions of each plan, all of which will be displayed clearly in a consistent format online so that you can easily compare "apples to apples." Exchange staff will be available to assist those who do not have online access, who need help understanding their options, or who need assistance navigating the system. You choose the company and level of coverage that you think will best serve your interests.

There are four possible levels of coverage for each person. You choose the level you can afford, given your health care needs. The Platinum Plan is most expensive but pays 90% of your total medical cost; the Gold model pays 80%; the Silver plan pays 70% and Bronze, the least expensive, covers 60% of your costs. There is an exception. A lower payout, but less costly Catastrophic Plan will be offered to persons under age 30.

The Affordable Care Act sets minimum policy standards for services that must be covered in every health plan. These guaranteed services—including annual health assessments, free vaccinations, mammograms and other women's health services—are a big part of keeping America healthy. Regulations and details about these minimums are still in development and will be finalized by HHS.

Once each year you as a customer can switch to a new policy within the same company or one with another provider. The rationale behind the exchange is to provide you with transparency and competition so you can have the best chance to get the policy that meets your needs at the best price. **You will never in your life face the prospect of going without basic health insurance that you can obtain at the lowest cost in the category you can afford.**

Health insurance companies have had the difficult task of setting limits on costs and treatment options. They have been criticized, fairly and unfairly, when they have placed limits on payments for overcharges and unnecessary procedures. However, rather than confronting escalating prices systematically, they have generally preferred to make payments to doctors, hospitals and other providers and simply pass along the costs by steadily raising premiums. The increased regulation of private insurance companies—limiting their profits, requiring minimum standards of coverage, requiring them to use standard claim forms, requiring them to present policy choices in a consistent, transparent way on competing exchanges, etc.—is one among many ways that the new law expects to save money for you the consumer and for the government.

Special Provisions Already in Effect

Most of the law goes into effect gradually, over several years. It will take time to set up systems, employ personnel and work through all of the agreements. Several aspects of the law are already in effect. Five provisions are already quite popular.

First, the Affordable Care Act provides that unmarried children up to age 26 can be covered on their parents' insurance plan. This is of immediate help to young adults who are out of school but have not found employment that provides health insurance. The provision is especially helpful at this time of high unemployment. The national rate of coverage increased from 66.1% to 69.6% between July 2010 and July 2011 and represents coverage for an additional one million young adults.[5] In addition, a special provision in the Medicaid section of the law provides coverage for foster care children who have graduated from the social service system because of age.

Second, the Act abolishes lifetime or annual limits on the amount an insurance company must pay for a needed service. In the past, a policy might say in the fine print that it would pay only a certain amount annually or a modest total amount during a lifetime for a designated illness. The Affordable Care Act eliminates the fine print and provides genuine security to many who have seen the safety rug pulled out from under them at a time of greatest need.

A third immediate benefit of the law is that beginning steps toward closing the Medicare "donut hole" have been put into effect. Before the ACA, Medicare would pay up to $2,840 within a year for prescription drugs. Beneficiaries were then required to pay 100% of their prescription costs above $2,840. But if the actual patient cost soared past $4,550, Medicare again assumed the payment. This break in coverage is called the "donut hole." Nearly four million Medicare beneficiaries were affected by this coverage gap in 2010. The first step in closing that hole in 2010 was to provide a $250 rebate to each person who fell in. By November, 2011 the donut hole had shrunk by 40% for those who landed in it. The average cost per patient in the donut hole fell from $1,504 in 2010 to $901 in 2011. A 50% discount on brand-name drugs secured from pharmaceutical companies yielded an average savings of $581 and Medicare picked up more of the cost of generic drugs, saving the remainder. The Pharmaceutical Research and Manufacturers of America agreed to the discount as part of an understanding with the White House when the bill was being written. The entire donut hole will be closed as additional reforms are gradually implemented over a period of ten years. This represents a major new benefit for older Americans.

A fourth program that went into effect in 2010 is the Early Retirement Reinsurance Program (ERRP). It offers affordable insurance for workers and their families who retire before age 65 because of illness or layoff. Employers join to protect their laid off workers. Unions, government agencies, or religious organizations with a large number of employees can join if they have been responsible for insurance. Insurance companies agree to reenroll retirees and provide lower cost for premiums, with the government offering subsidies. The first year ending December 31, 2010, 5,000 employers or contractors were enrolled into ERRP. They covered 61,000 early retirees at a cost of $535 million, according to a report released by HHS in June of 2011. Without this program individual insurance plans for persons in this age group would be prohibitively expensive for most.

The fifth, and perhaps the most humane aspect of the new law already in effect says that insurance companies cannot cancel your policy after you have an accident or develop a catastrophic illness. When President Obama signed the health care legislation in March 2010 he said at the ceremony, "Today, I am signing this reform bill into law on behalf of my mother, who argued with insurance companies even as she battled cancer in her final days." Heart-wrenching stories like that of the President's mother abound, telling of families who thought they were secure with health insurance, only to find their policies cancelled when a family member contracted a debilitating and expensive illness.

Senator Ron Johnson (R. Wisc.) wrote an op-ed[6] in *The Wall Street Journal* in which he described his daughter's emergency heart surgery many years ago as an argument against the Affordable Care Act. He wrote, "I don't even want to think what might have happened if she had been born at a time and place where government defined the limits for most insurance policies and set precedents on what would be covered." He continued, "Would the life-saving procedures that saved her have been deemed cost-effective by policy makers deciding where to spend increasingly scarce tax dollars?"

The new Senator won office based in part on his red-hot opposition to the health care law. In fact, he was blatantly distorting the truth. Mr. Johnson was a high official in a plastics company that provided a good policy. He was fortunate that the insurance company did not cancel his policy after emergency surgery determined his daughter had a preexisting condition which was not revealed when the policy was written. One wonders if an hourly worker on the assembly line would have been so fortunate. It is some insurance companies who ration care to increase their profits. This law eliminates that option and ensures that nobody will be denied care when it is most needed. In fact, everybody is covered. **This law is a hallelujah chorus bringing joy and new life for the 10,000 additional persons each year who were being kicked off their health insurance protection.**

Expanding to Underserved Populations

We will fall short of a healthy America until racial minorities and low income citizens have equal access to health care. These groups have limited access, and the quality of care they do get is markedly inferior. Blacks, Hispanics, and others who are financially distressed have a backlog of "deferred maintenance" that puts them even farther behind. For example, the infant mortality rate for African-Americans is twice the rate as that for non-Hispanics whites. The diabetes rate is nearly double. The list of such disparities is tragically long.

Care and compassion shine through the 1,000+ page ACA and many special programs target subgroups of underserved citizens. For example, The Children's Health Insurance Program (CHIP) is expanded and enriched with an initial 23% increase in federal funds. This program, like Medicaid, is funded jointly by federal and state dollars.

States will be required to provide a new level of service that meets minimum federal standards, including prescription drugs, dental and mental health services. The states may provide more services than those required, and they have the option to enroll persons up to 150% of the poverty line. The new law also includes funding to increase public awareness about CHIP. Many parents whose children are eligible for CHIP don't know it. Poorer states, especially in the south, have not made an effort to inform their citizens, as this would increase their costs. To be eligible for federal assistance, states must now introduce quality outreach programs to make sure the vulnerable are enrolled.

Medicaid requires even larger chunks of money from the federal and state treasuries than does CHIP. Medicaid has always enrolled select groups below the poverty line but the Affordable Care Act extends coverage to everyone below the poverty line, along with those whose incomes are up to 133% of the poverty line. States have the option to enroll persons up to 150% of the poverty level, as it may be more efficient to cover these people through Medicaid than through subsidized private insurance.

Medicaid enrollees include seniors on Medicare who are too poor to pay a share of their medical costs. Seniors' personal funds are often exhausted during the last years of life by illnesses and hospital stays. More than half of Medicaid costs are spent caring for frail elderly persons. These enrollees are called "dual eligibles" because they qualify for both Medicare (over 65) and Medicaid (impoverished). This small percentage of the population will always use a disproportionate amount of health funds, as illnesses tend to increase at the end of life.

Modifying the Health Care Delivery System

The law encourages the restructuring of our health delivery system. Our current system is primarily a "fee for service" structure. In other words, when I go for a physical exam my insurance company pays a fee with very few questions asked of the doctor. If my doctor says I need an x-ray, I may schedule an appointment at a hospital or radiology facility and get the films, which are interpreted by a specialist who sends a report back to my primary physician. The radiologist and my primary physician are both paid by the insurance company. When I go to the hospital I may be charged every time I take a pill or get my blood pressure checked by a nurse. The big costs come from the operating room. There my total bill is based on the number and types of procedures. These bills usually are paid without consideration of whether the procedures were necessary. The bottom line: both doctor and hospital get paid more if they perform more procedures and tests. This creates a culture of "quantity over quality" and discourages an integrated, patient-centered approach to care. Medicare and Medicaid patients whose bills are covered by government funds pay differently at the hospital. The inpatient expenses are rolled into a single reimbursement based on the diagnosis. Many states choose to place Medicaid patients into a pool and negotiate a single contract with an insurance company or other provider to meet their medical needs for a set fee. Also, some corporate hospital plans, and indeed, some private health insurance plans already pay a set fee for a hospital visit rather than "fee for service."

The Affordable Care Act nudges the nation toward a thoroughly revised delivery system, based on the recognition that the American health care system needs to be cured of its high spending and disorganized ways. One new structure for achieving this result is the Accountable Care Organization (ACO). An ACO may be formed by a hospital, a health insurance company or by a group of physicians. Most frequently, each health provider is paid a salary, although some restricted fees for services are possible. The group compensation is a set annual amount, based on the number of enrollees and the cost of treating that general population the year before the ACO was formed. Each ACO must enroll at least 5,000 persons. Facilities will typically include labs, eye care, pediatrics, maternity care, and other specialties, often in the same building. The group may have contracts with hospitals where they place their own surgeons, or they contract for the use of hospital surgeons.

The ACO health care providers have an incentive to lower costs because they share in the savings, using costs from the previous year as the baseline. They can save money by using electronic records. They can eliminate unnecessary tests, surgeries and prescription drugs. They focus on keeping clients well rather than just treating illnesses, because this, too, will save them money. We, the public, along with members of the ACO, share in the savings they create.

Major Emphasis on Wellness

The Affordable Care Act envisions every American having a primary care physician. Ideally, we become partners with our doctors as we come to know and trust each other in a long-term relationship. Through this partnership the patient becomes an educated consumer who understands healthy living. The doctor is expected to have electronic health records that document our medical histories. When we have appointments we use the time well to discuss our medical needs.

Many Americans now have such a professional relationship with a single doctor who guides them in health care. Unfortunately, far too many of us do not. When the Affordable Care Act is fully implemented, every American will have the opportunity to have a primary care provider who will also coordinate referrals to specialists. Every insurance policy is required to cover annual physicals and necessary inoculations with no copayment or additional charge to the patient.

The Affordable Care Act places major emphasis on wellness and preventive care. Think about it. If we live with good health we not only enjoy a fuller, more productive life, we also save on medical expense. Physicians will be trained to emphasize ways to enhance wellness and will be paid extra for achieving this. In the fee-for-service system their financial incentive is to treat illness, run tests, and do surgeries. Under the new system, a doctor may find it appropriate, for example, to inquire about the length of the workday for their patients, as recent research indicates that adults who work more than 11 hours a day have a 67% higher risk of developing coronary disease than those who work eight hours. Or, a doctor may test and monitor risk factors for diabetes or heart disease, so these can be addressed with preventive measures, counseling, and lifestyle changes before they become major health issues.

Employers will find it profitable to offer incentives to workers if they take steps to improve their health. Both management and workers will be recognized and rewarded for promoting good health. For example, a team of Harvard researchers published an article in the *Journal of Health Affairs* in 2010 reporting on their study of employer-sponsored fitness programs.[7]   The study showed that "medical costs fall by about $3.27 for every dollar spent on wellness programs and that absenteeism costs fall by about $2.73 for every dollar spent." Further, Medicare and Medicaid providers will be trained to work more effectively with patients on preventive health measures such as encouraging them to get proper exercise, eat a healthy diet, stop smoking, curb alcohol and drug abuse, get medical checkups, and take their prescribed drugs.

Obesity control is a big new challenge for this generation. The Affordable Care Act requires the phasing in of more complete food labeling for all products sold in grocery stores. It also mandates that calorie labels and nutritional information be on display for foods sold in restaurant chains with more than 25 outlets. Further, it promotes public advertizing to make citizens aware of unhealthy eating practices. Popular athletes and musicians will be enlisted to lead these programs.

A big national reversal is possible. We can become far healthier by learning to assume personal responsibility, nudged by programs that support good health. As an example, consider how we have lowered the level of smoking in America. Airlines in the 1950s, when a majority of American adults smoked, welcomed smoking anywhere in the passenger cabin. When we learned about secondhand smoke and some travelers expressed discomfort sitting next to a smoker, the airlines separated passengers into smoking and non-smoking sections. For several years the division of sections was about equal. Then as public awareness campaigns got under way and labeling of tobacco packages was mandated, more people stopped smoking. Eventually the smoking area shrank to about one-fourth of the aircraft passenger area. Finally, smoking on airplanes was outlawed. Today fewer than 20% of Americans smoke. They are often treated at work or in public buildings as renegades sent out into the heat or cold to smoke. **Better health can be achieved through public awareness! Hundreds of thousands of citizens live today because of these public awareness programs**.

Abortion Restrictions

The Hyde Amendment, passed on September 30, 1976, mandated that no federal funds be spent for abortions. This same policy was assumed from the beginning of the health care debate in Congress. Nonetheless, opponents of abortion wanted more explicit language in the bill to assure them that absolutely no federal money would go for that purpose.

The Bill was crafted so that insurance policies provided through the exchanges would not pay for any abortion services. However, families that felt the need for such coverage could add a rider, paid for separately, that would cover abortion services under specified circumstances. Page after page of the new law spells out in great detail how this service is bought, divorced from any policy the federal government supports or subsidizes. Some Democrats who strongly oppose abortion joined the

Republican ranks in opposing the entire legislation until they were satisfied with the wording on not covering abortion services. However, since the law's enactment abortion opponents continue to keep the issue alive. They are working through receptive state legislatures to remove abortion coverage from the insurance exchanges, even when it is paid for privately. Currently, more than 80% of insurance companies cover abortion services as part of their policies. They are now creating special policies just for this purpose and billing the customers separately. By April 2011, five states had passed laws forbidding insurance companies from providing abortion coverage even though no federal dollars are involved.

Some groups are opposed not only to abortion but also to birth control. Whereas most people see birth control as the most effective way to prevent abortion, the Roman Catholic Church in particular sees any method of population control other than sexual abstinence as anti-life. They object to being mandated to pay for insurance that includes birth control measures for employees in universities, hospitals, etc., even when non-Catholic employees seek this coverage. The Obama administration offered a compromise. Church-related organizations would not have to pay for contraceptive coverage, but employees could still receive free coverage if desired, paid for by the insurance company.

Women's rights organizations see the reproductive needs of women being systematically denied as the nation moves backward to a dark era of unwanted children and back-alley abortions. Those who are poor will be disproportionately affected. The Religious Coalition for Reproductive Choice comprises national organizations from major religious faiths.   They are now uniting to support reproductive choice and the option for those who need abortion coverage to get it with private funds through policies sold on the exchanges.

New Insurance Program for Late Life Costs

A new program, the Community Living Assistance Services and Support Act (CLASS) is established by the ACA to provide working Americans with optional long-term care insurance.   It is a self-financed government insurance program that does not cost the taxpayer money. This should be less expensive than private long-term care insurance, since the government will not be making a profit.   CLASS is slated to get under way in 2012.   The primary purpose is to help subscribers afford an assisted living facility if needed in later years or to continue living at home but with home health assistance.   This insurance will also benefit the government by keeping many seniors off the rolls of Medicaid.   The program is self-financed, like Social Security, with funds taken regularly from the paychecks of employees.   But this time the program is voluntary.   It provides a benefit up to $1,500 added income per month, so that Social Security combined with CLASS would be sufficient for most persons to afford the living assistance they may require.

Medicaid spends more than $103 billion annually on nursing home care, assisting the frail elderly and persons with disabilities.   It pays for nearly half of long-term care costs.   If enough people enrolled in CLASS, perhaps half or more of those billions can be saved by Uncle Sam, and the elderly would have more options and more control of their own health care and living situations late in life.

Note: On October 14, 2011 Health and Human Services Secretary Kathleen Sebelius announced her department had decided to dismiss CLASS. She stated that this part of the ACA is being placed on hold because it could not "be implemented in a workable fashion." The experts judged that not enough healthy people would sign up to make it financially self-supporting over a long period of time, even though it would run a surplus for the first ten years.

Critics of the ACA claimed this is one more proof that the entire law is fatally flawed. They have held Congressional hearings with the goal of passing legislation to strike CLASS from the law. Proponents say it demonstrates that the Obama administration has proved its willingness to cull the law's failures and it represented a moment of integrity in support of a strong law. Supporters pointed out that the national need for such insurance remains. Ms. Sebelius noted in her letter, "The challenge that CLASS was created to address is not going away." Only 2.8% of Americans have private long-term care coverage. By 2020 an estimated 15 million persons will need to cover such costs. When the elderly run out of money, they become eligible for Medicaid. Placing citizens on public care rather than self-financed private care is expensive for the state and federal governments. HHS is studying ways to revise the terms of CLASS in order to make it sustainable.

Overview Summary

This overview does not cover every feature of the new law but it does provide general information and some analysis of its primary provisions. The next three chapters will go into more detail about the three purposes of the law: to cover everyone, to improve the quality of our health care, and to lower costs. **One thing is abundantly clear: our old system is hopelessly broken. It would be a disaster to repeal the new health care law and return to the past.**

Chapter 2

UNIVERSAL COVERAGE

Among adults under age 65, 73% of those with private health insurance had excellent or very good health, compared with 55% of adults without health insurance.
—National Center for Health Statistics, Series 252, p. 42

Until March 23, 2010 when the Affordable Care Act was signed into law, at least 32 million Americans lived without health insurance. Most of these Americans feared illness, and in many cases death, without adequate health care. With no family doctor, they had access only to crisis care in the emergency room. The Affordable Health Care Act offers hope for deliverance.

Throughout the last quarter of the 20th century and into the 21st, the number of us without insurance accelerated like a car careening down a mountain road. The soaring cost of insurance was causing employers to cut back on benefits or eliminate insurance benefits entirely because they could no longer afford to cover the cost. Too many of the self-employed got priced out of the market. Just as significantly, many with "preexisting conditions" were barred by the insurance companies from ever receiving coverage again or had rates raised so high coverage became unaffordable. The working poor had no money left from living expenses to buy expensive health insurance.

The nation faced an enormous mess! The health insurance system could not be sustained. Only because we suffered so much and faced such economic chaos did we finally overcome the inertia of gridlock and deal with our dilemma. Only because some of us heard the cries of pain and loss did we join hands and hearts with other compassionate Americans to finally enact a national law supporting universal coverage.

Best and Worst States

Gallup released a survey in March 2011 showing the percentage of uninsured persons in each state. There is one state that has superior coverage by a large margin: Massachusetts. Massachusetts is the nation's best, the only state with a plan similar to the new national law. It was enacted during a Republican administration, when Mitt Romney was governor. Governor Romney deserves a hallowed place in national history for guiding the state through the enactment of this far-reaching and humane health care reform, charting a course for the nation's future.

States that provide the highest level of insurance coverage for its citizens are: Massachusetts, with only 4.7% uninsured; Connecticut, 9.9%; Minnesota, 10.5%; Hawaii, 10.6%; Pennsylvania, 11%; and Vermont, 11% uninsured. Texas and Louisiana share the dubious honor of having the highest percentage of uninsured persons, with 25% of residents without coverage. Florida dropped from 17.8% uninsured in 1999 to 22.4% in 2009. Generally, the "red" states in the south leave the most people facing illness and death without proper medical care.

Locating the Uninsured

The uninsured fall into six broad categories: (1) those in the process of changing jobs, (2) the working poor who cannot afford coverage, (3) those denied care because of pre-existing conditions, (4) those who can afford coverage but choose to ignore it, (5) nine million persons with annual incomes over $75,000 who choose to self-insure and can demonstrate they are qualified, and finally (6) citizens who live abroad. The Affordable Care Act of 2010 provides a new path leading to full coverage for 32 million of us, most being in the first four categories. We look more closely at these four groups of uninsured persons and see how the new law applies to them.

Those Changing Jobs

The new law makes it easier to change jobs without worrying about losing health insurance. This is important because 45% of Americans get their health plans through their employers and on the whole job turnover is high during the course of one's career. Businesses feel free to dismiss even good workers in order to increase profits. Likewise, workers often lack loyalty to their employers. High mobility is a hallmark of today's work place. Because health insurance benefits vary greatly from one business to another, the process of changing to a new provider in a new company has often been confusing and difficult. If a new health problem occurred, it would be considered a "pre-existing condition" by any future insurance company. It could be quite literally "the kiss of death" to change jobs.

Workers often feel trapped into staying with miserable jobs because they fear losing insurance. They have little assurance that a new job will provide them their same level of care. The sad truth is that many lose coverage completely when they change jobs and start over.

States regulate their health insurance systems with unique requirements in each state. Insurance companies, therefore, must tailor policies to people within a given state, making it difficult to transfer insurance policies across state lines. During the health reform debate, Republicans in the Senate claimed they could solve much of our health care problem by extending insurance policies across state lines, without the fundamental reforms of this law. That would seem hard to do, considering the often contradictory state structures. But under the new Affordable Care Act, with federal standards, employees of small companies will get a voucher from the employer and take it to a state exchange, where they will use it to buy insurance. Once each year they can change insurance companies or plans within a company. When they move to a different job, even in a different state, workers can easily arrange to begin coverage at the new exchange, if necessary. Larger employers must either provide insurance or give vouchers for employees to use at a state exchange. Every employer policy must meet basic standards.

Competitive bidding is limited when the pool of claimants is from a sparsely populated state. Now only one or perhaps two providers are typically willing to offer policies in a low population state. Those few companies can charge residents higher prices than in states where competition is keen. Under the new law, states are required to merge their insurance requirements with those of a neighboring state and combine insurance pools, if needed, in order to get enough enrollees to spread the risk while maintaining competition.

In these ways, the new law facilitates worker coverage at lower rates and makes it easier for most workers to change jobs without losing health insurance.

The Working Poor

The working poor are "caught between a rock and a hard place." People below the poverty line are covered by Medicaid. Our biggest remaining challenge is to cover those in the lower middle class, as the $25,000 to $49,000 income range has the highest percentage of people without health insurance. In today's market the cost of health insurance is so high that the working poor cannot afford it. The Affordable Care Act adjusts the cost of insurance on a sliding scale according to the worker's income. The subsidy is modest at 400% of poverty but much larger in the $25,000 to $49,000 income range.

Before the ACA was passed, Medicaid eligibility was at 100% of the poverty line and below. The new law expands Medicaid to include people whose income is from 100% to 133% of the poverty line. This income group is afforded a complete basic medical plan and states are required to enroll them. In the past, some states saved money on Medicaid by restricting benefits, but the new law makes it abundantly clear that states can no longer offer more restrictive coverage than that mandated in the federal law. Furthermore, state plans must now cover prescription drugs and mental health services. It should be noted that states can choose to expand Medicaid up to 150% of the poverty line and the federal government will pay its half of the cost between 133% and 150%. Finally, each state must submit an annual report to Health and Human Services giving full details on Medicaid enrollment and the level of services.

Case Study: A Working Married Couple

Nancy and Bill live modestly. They do not have children. It is evident that they care deeply for each other. Bill is a painter and is employed by a company that paints houses. Bill makes $15 per hour but is unemployed in bad weather and during part of the winter. Nancy works for a retail store and makes $12 an hour. She works 30 hours a week except during the Christmas holidays when her hours at work are as high as 50 per week.

One recent winter Nancy began to lose energy and feel increasingly lethargic. She pushed herself to stay on the job but then she would collapse on the couch when she got home from work. Bill was worried, as this was unusual behavior for Nancy. Unfortunately, they had no health insurance and neither ever saw a doctor. Bill decided they should spend $150 to get a medical diagnosis of Nancy's problem.

The doctor, after tests, sounded the alarm and ordered Nancy to the hospital for emergency surgery. Bill was distraught. He wanted Nancy home and her health restored. But he also realized they had no insurance and only limited savings, as they lived "month to month."

Nancy did recover. She came home after six days in the hospital, but they had a medical bill of $20,000. The hospital pushed Bill for payment. He depleted a savings account of $2,000 and added the $500 set aside for the next month's rent. Now they were saddled with a $17,500 debt, were a month behind on rent, and Nancy had to recuperate for a month before she could go back to work.

I know this couple. They rented their townhouse from me. They got behind another month on the rent. I hired Bill for a month's rent, to paint the interior of the house they were renting from me. After three months of financial struggle, they moved to live with Nancy's mother.

This is a familiar story. The hospital may lose most of the money owed to them. I lost two months' rent. They would have been forced into bankruptcy if there had been enough assets or income to make it worthwhile for the hospital to sue. Bill and Nancy are two of 16 million citizens who desperately need health insurance but go without because they simply can't afford it. Under the new law they will pay what they can and be covered by public funds for the remainder.

Pre-Existing Conditions

Recall the situation in our country before the Affordable Care Act passed in 2010. Five million persons, mostly in the middle class, faced a living nightmare. One day a person would be healthy and care-free with good health insurance. The next day he or she woke up to find a debilitating health problem that would only get worse. Then their health insurance company would look for pre-existing conditions and other loopholes to cancel the policy or raise the premiums so high they were unaffordable. Family finances drained away rapidly. Money was soon exhausted, as they paid for expensive prescription drugs and delicate operations. Once they lost their insurance policy they could not get another one because now they had a pre-existing condition. These neighbors and friends would have to get by without health insurance until they became eligible for Medicare at age 65.

In the past, health insurance companies realized that if they could demonstrate that a patient had a pre-existing condition that had gone unreported when the policy was awarded they could cancel that policy and save money. The old system left the decision about whether to cancel the policy to the same insurance company that would benefit from the cancellation. The door was open for abuse, and 10,000 patients a month lost their insurance this way. Let it be acknowledged that reputable insurers did not cancel policies unless the right to do so was written into the policy's fine print—the very, very fine print!

This same tragic reality confronted many parents with newborn babies. If the infant had some deformity or illness, the baby could never be insured. These parents faced a double tragedy. They expended the ultimate in physical and emotional energy in caring for a child 24 hours a day. At the same time, their financial resources were decimated.

This entire nightmare system has now changed. Beginning with passage of the Affordable Care Act in March 2010, it became illegal for health insurance companies to drop coverage because of a pre-existing condition no matter what the fine print said. Those who had been dropped were ordered restored, the cost of including high risk persons phased in gradually so as not to create an unmanageable hardship on the insurance companies. Insurance companies can make this generous concession because of the millions of new clients being added to their rolls. **It is impossible to express in words the sense of relief for persons faced with death and now given life, or those weighed down with an impossible financial burden that now have the weight lifted! For many, life and hope were reborn.**

The Young and the Reckless

Half of the 35 million without health insurance can actually afford at least a basic policy, but they choose to go uninsured. The young are singled out in the new law as a special category. Many of them feel a sense of invincibility. Most have not had serious health problems, so they are reluctant to spend scarce dollars on insurance. As a way to encourage them to buy coverage, the law provides them a special category to buy only limited catastrophic insurance, less than the bronze level that covers 60% of the cost. The category of eight million young adults, ages 18 to 26, is the only group permitted to settle for this limited coverage.

Many of these same young people, especially if they are students, have not yet entered the workforce and established health insurance there. A provision went into effect in 2010 permitting them to get full coverage on their parents' policies until they finish school and/or find gainful employment that offers insurance. Beginning in 2014 children between ages 19 through 25 can stay on their parents' policy even if they are offered coverage from an employer. The special benefit applies for both married and unmarried children. The new law has already had a significant impact on coverage in this group of 29.7 million young adults.

The "reckless" make up the remainder. They expect to beat the odds. They bet they won't contract a debilitating illness, require an operation, or fall prey to a serious accident. If that should happen, they hope for enough money in the bank to pay the cost. Too often, it doesn't work like that in the real world. Too many lose to the odds when a serious illness or accident strikes. Uninsured people of every age group and economic level may find themselves in the hospital with huge medical bills. Providers then end up empty-handed and the unfortunate risk-takers are bankrupt. In addition, workers who do carry insurance pay higher premiums to make up the difference.

Everybody needs insurance. We all need it to protect our personal health and assure our financial wellbeing. In addition, the practical economic reality is that in order for our health care system to function effectively, everybody must have insurance.

The Affordable Care Act mandates that the reckless buy insurance. The Act speaks forcefully of "shared responsibility." It reminds us that under the old system those with coverage must pay the hospital bills for those without insurance. Why? Encased in a law signed by President Ronald Reagan—The Emergency Medical Treatment and Active Labor Act of 1986—is our national commitment not to let any citizen suffer and die without medical care when there is an emergency. Hence, hospitals are forbidden by law from turning away patients who arrive on their door steps without insurance. Private hospitals cannot "dump" these patients at public hospitals. Yet, the system permits the hospitals to recover most of the costs by raising premium prices on the rest of us. **Each** person with insurance pays on average an extra $1,000 a year to make up for the free ride of others.

The Insurance Mandate

Shared responsibility is a central theme of the law: individuals, insurance companies, hospitals, medical providers, drug companies and others are all challenged to bear their share of the responsibility to provide good health care for all people at an affordable price. Personal responsibility is a traditional Republican rallying cry. One would think they would embrace the concept here, rather than try to declare the law unconstitutional. Actually, Republicans won concessions during the debate over the law by insisting that the penalty for failing to obtain insurance should be lowered significantly. Beginning in 2014, after a month of non-compliance, a tax of $95 will appear on the person's federal income tax return. The amount is raised to $350 in 2015. The tax rises to $750 in 2016 and thereafter it is revised annually, based on cost of living adjustments.

Lawsuits have been filed by state attorneys general in 24 states challenging the constitutionality of forcing citizens to buy insurance against their wills. We need to be clear—the lawsuits do not challenge the law as a whole, only the "mandate" to require the purchase of insurance.

The Act predicts this pushback and makes a case for its mandate by explaining that it is covered by the interstate commerce clause in the Constitution. Clearly insurance is commerce and an entire system of commerce is contained in the Act. Millions of persons are priced out of the insurance market because of high prices, so government has an interest in solving a civic problem. One significant part of high cost occurs when "freeloaders" get insurance on their way to the hospital. Another is when they use health services without paying for them.

The Law School Dean at Liberty University, Matthew Staver, argued before the Fourth Circuit Court of Appeals in Richmond in an early lawsuit that not purchasing insurance is not commerce. He conceded that it would be best for each person to have insurance but insisted the government has no right to force it on reluctant citizens. He used an analogy, saying we should not force people to eat broccoli because it is good for you. Neal Katyal, Acting Solicitor General, countered that there is a national crisis in health care. The government has devised a plan of shared responsibility, necessary to meet a critical national need. Since almost everybody must use health services at one time or another, the issue is who will pay the cost.

The insurance industry was willing to accept the new law because of the argument that they will gain an additional 32 million enrollees. They reached an informal understanding with the White House to accept a cap on overhead and profit, lower their fees, cover people with preexisting conditions, etc., in return for this large pool of new customers. Much of the cost containment structure established in the law would unravel if we were to take back the mandate that everybody have health insurance coverage.

Some who support this mandate liken it to the requirement that everybody with a car must purchase automobile liability insurance. But opponents point out that nobody has to own an automobile. Others compare the mandate to social security insurance where every working person is required to pay into the program and every person receives benefits after retirement. The bottom line is that if a person wants the system to pay for his or her accident or illness, that person must contribute to the cost. **A free ride for the financially able is unacceptable.**

Establishing the State Exchanges

How can the Affordable Care Act address the need to create a more rational, fairly priced, well-functioning integrated system with universal care? How can it incorporate those whose medical expenses are paid by the federal or state governments? How can it shape the health care systems to meet regional needs, while agreeing on a fundamental philosophy of shared responsibility? These critical questions guided legislators as they crafted the Affordable Care Act and built a comprehensive system. Establishing state exchanges to facilitate insurance coverage is a necessary component of an integrated system. These exchanges provide a mechanism for millions of additional citizens to get health insurance.

The Act requires a comprehensive health insurance exchange to serve as an online marketplace in each state. States are being awarded grants to set up their exchanges during 2011 and 2012. While the Act provides guidelines and requirements, it allows the states considerable leeway to decide how their exchanges should be structured. 2011 was the year when state legislatures were expected to pass laws creating their comprehensive plans. Ideally, 2012 is the year to write regulations, and 2013 is the time to employ most staff, get office space, bring on-line the computer infrastructure system and train workers in preparation for the implementation phase beginning January 1, 2014. If a state has not made appropriate progress toward setting up its exchange or if willful non-compliance becomes evident, ACA authorities will set up the exchange and manage it on behalf of the state.

As with any major policy change, there is reluctance, uncertainty, and fear about whether this is good policy and whether it will work. Trouble is brewing in some state legislatures. Republicans gained control of many of these legislatures in 2010; they are split between traditional Republicans and Tea Party activists. Both groups see implementation as a road to "bureaucratic medicine" and they want nothing to do with it. The split is over whether to back away completely with the hope that President Obama will be defeated in 2012 so they can repeal the entire law, or whether to go ahead and design a state system more to their liking than the one that would be sent from Washington. For these state legislatures, both crafting their own version and accepting the federal version are bad choices.

The ACA gives the Secretary of Health and Human Services regulatory authority to establish national criteria for qualified health plans and to approve the state exchanges within these basic federal guidelines. HHS will:

- Assure that marketing plans aim for complete enrollment, including persons with significant health problems,
- Ensure significant choice in each exchange, including at least one non-profit provider,

- Make sure plans include all eligible low-income persons,
- Meet accreditation standards for all medical and clinical personnel and facilities,
- Provide adequate information to enrollees, available online,
- Oversee a rating system at each benefit level, based on price, quality and enrollee satisfaction,
- Provide assurance of complete computerized records of the exchange and its enrollees,
- Have the authority to certify, decertify, and recertify insurance companies.

These are basic requirements states must address when they create their exchanges. In areas where a state is not in compliance, the Department of Health and Human Services will offer assistance to help the state reach compliance. Beginning in 2017, states may propose innovative plans, as long as they meet all basic objectives of the system. Innovative models are encouraged to constantly upgrade the system. New models are designed to function for 10 years with evaluations along the way.

Large Employers

Employers with more than 200 workers must automatically enroll new full-time employees in a health insurance plan but not necessarily in an exchange. 95% of employers with over 50 employees provided insurance as of June 2011. Any employer with more than 50 workers who does not offer minimum bronze coverage must pay the exchange $2,000 per year per full-time employee, except for the first 30 employees, who are exempt. In businesses that do offer insurance to most of their employees, any employees not covered will then be required to purchase insurance through the exchanges. For these employees, the penalty to the company becomes $3,000 for each of the uninsured, or $750 for every employee of the company, whichever is less. All employer penalties go toward paying insurance in the exchange for those employees not covered by the employer, reducing the amount they pay out of pocket. Of course, offering superior insurance in a competitive market will help a firm attract good personnel and make for a happy work force.

Some large companies reward their high level executives lavishly with "Cadillac" insurance policies. The ACA imposes a new excise tax on any corporate plan with an annual premium above $8,500 for single coverage, and $23,000 for a family of four. The tax is 40% of the amount above the maximum plan on the exchange. The tax is designed to help pay the cost of bringing the uninsured into the system, but it also discourages lavish coverage.

Large employers, as a whole, support the new law. They recognize it as their best hope for containing soaring health costs that reduce profits. When they move their operation to an exchange, they can also streamline their own Department of Human Resources, as they are relieved of much of the responsibility for choosing an insurance company and then assisting employees with their policies. In the past, 86% of large employers offered policies through only one insurance company, or a corporation self-insured its personnel. They may continue these policies, but over time more companies may move to the exchange and permit employees to choose from several insurance providers, a plus for company employees.

Small Businesses

Small business is not rigidly defined in the Act, so there is some variation in the cut-off sizes of businesses to which specific provisions apply. For purposes of the exchanges, businesses up to 100 employees are part of the program known as the Small Business Health Options Program (SHOP). Yet, states have the option to limit this program to businesses with up to 50 employees.

Businesses with fewer than 50 employees are exempt from the requirement to provide health insurance for employees. However, they may opt to offer insurance at a reasonable cost through the SHOP program. Incentives are provided that make it hard to resist. Businesses with 25 employees or fewer, with employee average annual incomes of not more than $40,000, are eligible for a tax credit of up to 35%, if they pay for at least 50% of the cost of premiums. Beginning in 2014 they can receive a two year tax credit of up to 50% of the premiums. For businesses with between 26 and 50 employees, the government will pay 25% of the insurance cost. This special assistance is offered to smaller firms who make limited profits, or who are just getting started in business. Currently, fewer than half of these small firms offer health insurance to employees. **The exchange system is an enormous benefit to these small businesses across the country and will strengthen them and the economy over time.**

We turn now to the insurance programs sponsored by the federal government. Created over time, they now stand alongside private insurance provided through employment. The public programs provide health care for

25.3% of the population. Each of these government programs has been evaluated, strengthened and incorporated into the Affordable Care Act.

Medicare

The most significant government health-related program in size and cost is Medicare. Medicare already provides universal coverage for all older Americans. Citizens and their employers pay into the Medicare insurance program throughout their working lives and are then eligible to receive coverage at age 65. Some 48 million recipients are now enrolled and the number is growing rapidly as "baby boomers" retire. Medicare cost $519 billion in 2010 and is growing as more citizens reach age 65 and as costs continue to rise out of control. The cost per year is projected to be $929 billion by 2020.

Some opponents of Medicare characterize it as a "government handout," ignoring the fact that workers have paid into the insurance pool throughout their working lives. Nonetheless, costs of services and the types of medical care now available have pushed the costs upward to the point where, even with the cost containment measures currently in place as a result of the ACA, Medicare costs are expected to exceed payments into the system by 2021 or sooner. And by 2029 if not sooner the Medicare Trust Fund will be able to cover only 85% of expenditures rather than 100%. These unsustainable cost projections provided part of the rationale for why the Affordable Care Act was created and signed into law. Obviously, even more work needs to be done in order to achieve long-term sustainability of the Medicare Trust Fund.

Lyndon Johnson signed the Medicare bill into law on July 30, 1965. At that time **51% of seniors had no medical insurance and 30% of seniors lived in abject poverty.** **Today virtually 100% have medical care and only 7% live in poverty.** **What a difference Medicare and Social Security have made!** According to a 2011 Associated Press poll 84% of those over age 65 said Medicare is "very important" to their well-being. 72% of all adults in the same poll said Medicare is "extremely important" or "very important" for their retirement security.

Medicare Part A is available for all persons age 65 and over who have been in the work force and to more than 7.8 million disabled persons. Medicare Part A provides insurance to cover stays in the hospital and in skilled nursing facilities, but not for long-term nursing home, in home, or assisted living care. Medicare Part B is optional and cost a patient in 2011 between $110 and $115 per month. Part B covers doctors' services and outpatient care. Also included are physical and occupational therapy and some home health care. This part of the package is designed to cover 80% of the total cost of these items. Many seniors take supplemental insurance to pay the balance. Prescription drug coverage (Medicare Part D) began in 2006. Medicare is financed by a payroll tax of 2.9%, divided equally between employer and employee.

Medicaid

Medicaid is a "means tested" insurance program for persons with low incomes and limited resources. The program was created at the same time as Medicare and was signed into law in July of 1965 as Title XIX of the Social

Security Act. Each state administers its own program and pays half the costs, while the federal Center for Medicare and Medicaid Services (CMS) establishes responsibilities, eligibility standards, quality of medical care and other criteria. As with private insurance, payment is sent directly to the health care provider rather than to the enrollee. A child may be eligible for Medicaid even if the parent is an undocumented immigrant and hence not eligible. A glaring problem is that only four out of ten adults with incomes under the poverty line, qualifying them for Medicaid, are actually enrolled. The new law opens Medicaid to all poor people up to 133% of the poverty line and requires states to implement outreach programs to eligible people who are not yet enrolled.

Some states have chosen different names for their Medicaid programs. California uses Medi-Cal, Massachusetts calls its program MassHealth and Tennessee, TennCare. States usually bundle administration of Medicaid with the Children's Health Insurance Program (CHIP). Programs are administered in a variety of ways. In some states contracts are made directly with doctors, hospitals and other medical providers. In more than 60% of states, enrollees are served under contract with private providers in a "managed care" arrangement. A set amount is paid by the state per year per enrollee to a managed care company that, in turn, provides all needed medical care.

Dental services have long been mandatory for children, but states have had the option of whether to include adults. Now, under the Affordable Care Act, all enrollees in Medicaid are to receive full dental care.

One of the largest growth areas in Medicaid costs comes when seniors exhaust their resources and transition from Medicare to Medicaid. Many elderly persons spend their final days or years in a nursing home and 60% of these beds are occupied by Medicaid enrollees. Medicaid covers all of the costs for the elderly poor, except that Social Security income received by the enrollee is transferred to the nursing home. Most states permit each person to keep $66 per month from their Social Security income for personal expenses.

Medicaid has become very expensive for states and the federal government. Medicaid spending by the federal government was $204 billion in 2008, matched by similar outlays in the states. Medicaid now requires as much as 20% of the budgets of some states, and the percentage is growing. In addition, the recession of 2008-2010 led to a substantial increase in enrollments in most states. Nine states had an increase of 15% or more. Signs of improved employment lead planners to expect a gradual drop in the number of Medicaid enrollees.

Children's Health Insurance Program (CHIP)

With medical care out of reach for the low income population as a whole, Republicans and Democrats agreed that at least the children should be covered. The awful truth is that one in five children in America lives below the poverty line. All of these children should, in theory, be covered by Medicaid. In addition, many others whose family income is above that line are undernourished and medically undertreated. Children's Health Insurance Program (CHIP) was born in the 1997 and grew rapidly to a fifty-state program that covered 5 million children. In the next ten years the program spent $20 billion in federal funds, matched by state money and administered by the states. Each state defines its own program within broad federal guidelines.

The U.S. Census Bureau in 2007 found 8.1 million uninsured children who needed coverage. CHIP was extended until 2009, when it was reauthorized and expanded until 2013. President Obama said at the legislative signing, "This is a down payment on my commitment to cover every single American." CHIP was further improved in the Affordable Care Act. It is designed to assure medical care for all qualified children, without reference to the legal status of their parents. The new law expands federal funding for CHIP by 23% and extends the legislation until 2015. Another small innovation added to CHIP provides quality hospice care for poor children in both CHIP and Medicaid.

Military Insurance

This brings us to the military, the last major category for which the government provides health care. Advocates for the military insist it is "earned" not "given." Active duty service personnel receive any and all needed medical care as part of their compensation for service. Veterans have access to VHA hospitals and out-patient treatment for the rest of their lives. Medical service providers are all on salary, paid by Uncle Sam. This is the only part of our total system that could be labeled "socialist," if anyone felt the need to do so, since the government provides services directly by its own employees, rather than just paying private providers. On the other hand, TRICARE, the program for families of service personnel, pays most of the cost of insurance through private providers.

Covering Citizens in Underserved Areas

There is more to universal coverage than insurance. Even in this modern era there are underserved areas where access to doctors and hospitals is limited. Generally, inner cities have fewer doctors, hospitals and other health facilities and rural areas are even more underserved because they are spread out and hard to reach. In these areas, getting to a doctor's office may require miles of driving and it is often even farther to a hospital. Also, the Affordable Care Act designates "frontier areas," mostly along our southern border or in high density ethnic areas with strategies to improve access to care. At every point medical needs on American Indian reservations are specifically considered. The federal government subsidizes the cost of medical education for those who agree to work in one of these underserved areas for a given number of years. Funds are allotted for additional community hospitals and advanced medical equipment. Funds are provided for patients to be flown by helicopter, as required, to more advanced hospital facilities at a greater distance. Video and telephone communication systems will be put in place to increase contact with health providers. Every effort is made to overcome the barriers to universal coverage, with access to the full range of health care.

A Final Charge

Before this law passed, costs were soaring and care was inefficiently provided. Universal coverage was an impossible dream. For the first time the nation has a

vision that has been translated into a broad plan to provide health care for everyone. By 2019 the new law will extend insurance coverage to an additional 32 million Americans, roughly the population of Canada. **The huge challenge remains for people everywhere to support the Affordable Care Act and participate in making it a practical reality.** Universal coverage can come only through federal legislation, as government is the only entity large enough to make it happen. Let us hold the vision of health care for every person as the sacred obligation of our common humanity.

Chapter 3

QUALITY HEALTH CARE

The United States ranks 42th in lowest infant mortality rate, down from 12th in1960 and 21st in 1990.
> —World Health Organization, August 31, 2011

Life expectancy at birth in the US is an average of 78.14 years, which ranks 47th in highest total life expectancy compared to other countries.
> —CIA Factbook, 2008

Can the Affordable Care Act improve our nation's health? Yes, in dozens of ways when the law is fully implemented.

Some members of Congress argue that we have "the best doctors and hospitals in the world." We already have health care "about as good as it can get" and hence this new health law is unnecessary.

Consider the other side. Yes, we have advanced medical research and promising new pharmaceuticals. Yes, we have many world-renowned doctors and top-tier state-of-the-art hospitals. Yes, Members of Congress who make speeches critical of the ACA have access to the best quality care our nation provides. But the bad news is our system has excluded many people from continuing care.

Does anyone want to argue that the sixteen million persons who are too poor to pay for health insurance are receiving quality care, even though they do have access to the emergency room? And, for purposes of our current chapter, **we must also recognize the sad truth that even those who have good coverage and access to health care have poorer health outcomes than those achieved in other countries. This is unnecessary, indeed unacceptable, and the ACA addresses poor medical outcomes in various ways.**

Another factor influencing quality of health outcomes is that nobody monitors and manages the system as a whole. No independent body has been responsible for correcting shortcomings, exposing doctors who routinely make poor medical decisions, dealing with the gaps in service, or giving proper emphasis to using "best practices." Our hospitals and our doctors, on a whole, are not nearly as good as they can or should be. Provisions for women's special health care needs have never been adequately implemented. There is more bad news. Our country spends far more per person on health care than any other country in the world. Yet our health quality and outcomes are generally not nearly as good as they could be. We have a long way to go. The Affordable Care Act provides a roadmap.

Some people who benefit from the finest health service oppose the new law because they believe it benefits only the poor and the marginal at their expense. Their cold calculation leads them to fight for their perceived self-interest and therefore oppose the Affordable Care Act. These folks would do well to appreciate the many ways it will, in fact, also improve **their** health.

Let's face it. Our health care system is broken and needs this major overhaul. The new law will help us all. We will improve America's health simply by increasing the number of people with access to insurance. But beyond that, **the Affordable Care Act includes a myriad of built-in, targeted ways to improve health outcomes for everyone.** This chapter will highlight many important examples.

Electronic Medical Records

Moving medical records from paper to computer will help us reach each of the three goals of the new law: universal coverage, better health for all, and lower cost. We have a winner when we achieve three for the price of one! Here we focus on how electronic medical records contribute to good health outcomes. How will electronic records help?

Electronic records are easy to read and help eliminate medical error. Hand written prescriptions from doctor to pharmacist, for example, are often hard to read. The person filling the prescription may have to guess what it says. Each day at the hospital the doctor writes instructions for the nurses to follow as they treat the sick. Each day those reading the orders must decipher the notes. When instructions are on the screen they can be displayed at the nurses' station and, at the same time, in the patients' room in easy-to-read form. Alerts can be given electronically when it is time to take the next medicine. Medical records are kept automatically. There are tens of thousands of inadvertent mistakes each year due to hand-written instructions that are hard to read and pieces of paper that are lost. Many of these mistakes cost health and even life.

Electronic records can track the prescription drugs of non-hospital patients. Many people take far more drugs than they need. Often the family doctor is unaware of the number and kind of medications taken by her client. According to an article in *Consumer Reports on Health*, "The percentage of Americans taking five or more prescription medications almost doubled between 2000 and 2008, according to government statistics.... The older the person, the more likely he or she was taking five or more medications. Research has found that the chance of having an adverse drug event is 13% among people taking two medications but 82% for those taking seven medications." The Report states that one of the most important priorities for an annual checkup for patients on prescription drugs is to review everything they are taking, including over-the-counter drugs, vitamins, herbal remedies, eye drops, etc. About 60% of those taking as many as five drugs have at least one that is unnecessary and often harmful. The physician is in a far better position to monitor and adjust these drugs and other remedies as needed over time when they are tracked by computer.

An elderly woman I know who lives in an assisted living facility went to see her physician. She was having a negative reaction to her medicine. In searching for the reason, the doctor checked her daily regimen of drugs. To the surprise of family and doctor they found that the nurse gave her 13 pills each day. A few were left over from her doctor at the facility where she had lived previously. She had been in the hospital, and doctors there prescribed medicine she was still taking, unbeknown to her physician.

She was taking one prescription drug her current doctor thought he had told the nurse at the assisted living home to stop using. The friend remarked and the doctor tacitly agreed, "All of these drugs are enough to kill a young person, much less one 94 years old." Her problem cleared when she dropped several counterproductive drugs. A list of her prescription drugs would have flashed on the screen each time she came into the doctor's consultation room, if her medical records had been computerized, following her from hospital to assisted living home and outpatient doctor.

Much testing and lab work is redundant because of paper records. A patient has radiology films made in the offices of her general practitioner. She is told to see a specialist. The films are sent by mail, but have not caught up with the specialist when she arrives at his office. The specialist duplicates the scans, despite the health risk. Computer records transfer information at the speed of light and make one wonder how we managed with paper records and "snail-mail."

The transition to electronic records is progressing steadily, yet there are immediate barriers to implementation. Doctors have thick folders with papers for each visit made. It is expensive to transfer all of this information to electronic files. Even more daunting is the task of convincing many older doctors that "an old dog can learn new tricks." Some complain they don't know which computers and programs to buy, or how to use a computer efficiently.

By 2011 about 20% of hospitals had converted to electronic data and 30% of office-based primary care doctors had made the leap. We now have a total of 40,000 physicians who use 21st century standards! Most of even these doctors will need to upgrade their systems to comply with federal records requirements, as everyone moves to a system that is standardized, simple and comprehensive.

It will cost doctors, on average, $50,000 each to get fully digitized. The Affordable Care Act provides some $27 billion over the next ten years to encourage doctors and hospitals to go electronic. More than 500,000 doctors, dentists and nurse practitioners qualify for federal funds. Initial funding was part of the 2009 economic stimulus package. Doctors who have a specified percentage of Medicare and Medicaid patients will find a further inducement to cooperate. They can also receive funds through Medicare and Medicaid to complete their transition to digital records.

Sticks as well as carrots are embedded in the law. Starting in 2015, those medical providers who are not digital will have lower reimbursement rates. Cuts start with Medicaid, then Medicare and finally, all providers will be penalized when they seek reimbursement from insurance companies or Uncle Sam using paper records.

Patients' Understanding of their Drugs

About 90 million adults in the United States misunderstand at least some of the instructions on prescription drug labels, according to the Institute of Medicine. The Food and Drug Administration has found that only 75% of the leaflets included with prescriptions meet the agency minimum recommended criteria for usefulness. Tiny print, technical language and incomplete instructions are thought to play a role in the estimated 500,000 preventable out-patient medication errors that occur nationally each year. The drugs we take can have fatal side effects if we do not recognize the symptoms of adverse reaction and act on them immediately. *Consumer Reports* staff members went to several leading retailers of drug prescriptions and found that each company had a different description of the same drug, presented in a different way. Uniform labeling of instructions in easy to read format, as required in the new law, can save lives and improve health.

Reduce Hospital Errors

There is no national system for monitoring or reporting the number of preventable injuries and deaths in hospitals. A widely cited study in 2000 by the Institute of Medicine titled "To Err is Human" estimated that 98,000 persons each year die as a result of hospital errors. An updated article in the April 2011 issue of *Health Affairs* concludes that despite a decade of study and focus on the problem, "medical errors and other adverse events" occur in one-third of hospital admissions.

Hospital errors can include (a) failure to give a patient the right medication at the right time, (b) failure to monitor or stabilize a patient's condition, (c) a mistaken diagnosis, (d) failure to refer a patient to an appropriate specialist, (e) surgery on the wrong person or the wrong body part, or (f) most common, infections from failure to follow best hygiene procedures. Patients are at risk of developing severe infections when they are placed in intensive care rooms, for example, that were not cleaned properly after previously being occupied by patients with infectious diseases. Hospital infections are often spread when personnel do not wash their hands between patients.

The most egregious error occurs when the patient gets an inappropriate operation. A four year old boy has an operation on the wrong eye, or someone who needs a leg amputated has the wrong one cut off, leaving him without a good leg. According to *Kaiser Health News*,[8] seven years after a national protocol was put into place requiring mandatory rules to prevent operations on the wrong patient or body part, the problem has not improved. Safety experts say it may be getting worse. Joint Commission officials estimate that wrong-site surgery occurs 40 times a week in US hospitals and clinics. Dr. Mark Chassin, president of the Joint Commission since 2008, thinks such errors are growing in part because of increased time pressures. Eliminating these errors is more complicated than anyone had previously thought. Many doctors prize their independence and give only lip service to the list of steps that are supposed to be taken before an operation begins. Until the doctor makes sure he has the right patient or is operating on the right leg by going through protocols—like a pilot's safety check before takeoff—the numbers are not expected to improve. Medicare has announced it will no longer pay for such operations, and beginning in 2012 Medicaid is no longer compensating doctors and hospitals. That may be the ultimate weapon in the war against carelessness.

The Affordable Care Act confronts this looming problem of hospital error. First, it requires hospitals to establish protocols to monitor quality based on patient computer records. The protocol includes an analysis of the number of added hospital days caused by staff error. It is especially keen on tracking readmissions in the days immediately following discharge of patients. It monitors the number of deaths and the causes. Second, these reports are made transparent on a hospital's web site. The hospital is publically graded and its record is compared with that of others in the same state or metropolitan area. Perhaps most important from the hospital administration perspective, payment for procedures will be lowered for hospitals with below average records and increased for those that are superior.

The Joint Commission, which provides accreditation for hospitals, issued its first listing of "top performers" in September, 2011. Hospitals were rated on how well they followed recommended protocols for treating five of the most common challenges they face with their patients: quick response to heart attack, following proper heart failure protocols, treating pneumonia, preventing surgical infection, and dealing with children's asthma. Hospitals were judged, for example, on how often they gave aspirin on arrival to heart attack patients, gave pneumonia and flu vaccines appropriately or provided proper treatment to prevent blood clots. 405 hospitals were given top ratings. None of the prestige hospitals, such as Johns Hopkins, Mayo Clinic or Massachusetts General, made the grade. Many of the "left out" hospitals are taking immediate steps to upgrade their systems and get on the list next year. The process is beginning to work!

The Federal Aviation Administration regulates the aviation industry so that thousands of people per day safely fly around the country and around the world. Yet in the health care field, we have been tolerating deaths from medical errors of various kinds equivalent to a fully

loaded jumbo jet crashing every day.[9] **The Affordable Care Act is reducing this unacceptable level of avoidable medical errors.**

Restructuring Health Care Delivery

Community Health Centers (CHC) now provide primary care in medically underserved areas, mostly rural. Middle class persons with good insurance may be unaware of the existence of CHCs, since they generally target clients who are low-income and uninsured.   The Community Health Centers have grown in importance over the years as the number of uninsured persons has steadily increased. They are considered highly successful, and the Affordable Care Act infuses $11 billion, plus $2 billion from stimulus funds, into the CHC budget to upgrade and expand this system.   By 2015, the number of CHCs is expected to double to about 2,200 around the country. The Centers accept Medicaid and Medicare clients in addition to the uninsured.   While they welcome patients with private insurance plans, CHCs were designed primarily to serve the poor.

Those who wrote the ACA used the existing Community Health Centers as models and then expanded their number and the services they offer. The Act provided $1.5 billion for renovation of existing Centers and $9.5 billion to create new Centers in medically underserved areas.   The Centers provide a "medical home" and complete health care services to enrollees. Each enrollee has coordinated care with at least five specific services. These include (1) same-day or next-day appointments, (2) off-hours clinical advice by telephone, (3) tracking of test results and follow up to see that necessary services are carried out, (4) referring patients to specialists as needed and (5) prevention-oriented functions.   Not all of the existing 1,100 Centers now offer all of these services, but they will as they implement the Affordable Care Act. They offer medical homes, with a full array of services, to the poor who have been relegated to the fringes of health care. For millions of citizens who use Community Health Centers, both access and quality of health care are markedly improved over the era when the Centers did not exist.

The Accountable Care Organization

The Community Health Center has a cousin called the Accountable Care Organization (ACO).   An ACO is often a large organized group of family practice and specialist physicians and support personnel closely associated with a hospital. The core concept is that the ACO agrees to provide a medical home for people of all economic strata who live in a particular geographic area. The Affordable Care Act sets 5,000 as the minimum number of clients needed to form an ACO.

How are ACOs expected to improve quality of services delivered? Providers receive an annual fee that includes all services for each enrollee based on prior costs. They receive bonuses by delivering better health results for less than past costs. The Congressional Budget Office estimated that the ACO program will save Medicare alone some $5 billion through 2019, while eliminating the problem of physicians not wanting to take Medicare patients because of being paid lower than standard fees.

Quality of care is monitored. The law originally proposed 65 standards by which quality will be judged. They fall into five areas: (1) the team's effectiveness in treating the medical problems of patients, (2) how the patients feel about the experience of care, (3) the extent to which care is coordinated, (4) patient safety, and (5) the degree of emphasis on preventive health. On October 20, 2011 the Administration announced a revised set of standards, reducing the number of quality measures that ACOs must meet from 65 to 33.

ACOs provide comprehensive care. Case managers visit in the homes of the elderly and disabled to assess changing needs and appropriate services. ACO home health aides may assist with daily living tasks, such as dressing, bathing, grooming, taking medications and perhaps preparing some hot meals. They promote wellness programs. They coordinate hospital stays and see that medical instructions are followed when enrollees return home from the hospital. The more ways they can help sustain wellness and effectively manage illness, the larger will be the rewards for those who work in the ACO. This financial incentive will also discourage unnecessary tests, procedures, and prescriptions that now for the first time will cost money to those who order them.

Private insurance companies like Humana, United Health Group, WellPoint and Aetna are all moving to set up ACOs. Why? They have much to gain by containing costs. However, red flags need to be raised. The barrier between companies that provide insurance and those that provide care is crumbling. These giant insurance companies could gain even greater control over our health care system if they are permitted to set rates that protect their profits while controlling physicians and deciding which medical procedures to use and which doctors to employ.

The Community Health Centers will serve more dispersed populations and areas where there is a concentration of low income persons or senior citizens. In contrast, ACOs are more likely to be established in highly populated cities and serve a wide economic cross-section of clients.

Medical Homes

The Affordable Care Act includes development money, administered through the states, to set up a new system of "medical homes." Community Health Centers and ACOs already provide medical homes for their clients. However, other organizations will also utilize the medical home model. Medicaid will be one of the first to implement it. In the medical home model, treatment is coordinated by a primary care physician who maintains an on-going relationship with patients. However, the doctor is supported by information technology and a team of health professionals.

A key member of the team is the non-physician care manager who guides patients to proper medical services, including hospitals, home health agencies and nursing homes. This care manager also has training as a health coach who provides information and encouragement for good eating habits, exercise and other wellness efforts. Pilot projects have demonstrated that the medical home system can greatly reduce hospitalizations and emergency room visits. The system substantially cuts costs, and for our purposes here, improves the quality of care by providing an important new level of monitoring and support for vulnerable persons.

Case Study: the VHA and Quality Care

Right here in our own country, the Veterans Health Administration gives us a shining example of a major turnaround in our nation's largest integrated health care system. Over the past ten to twenty years, the VHA has been remade into arguably the best health care system in the United States in terms of quality, using many of the same measures we have been discussing.

In the early 1990s, the VA hospitals were in a state of disarray, with dilapidated facilities, poor quality care, and a rigid, inefficient bureaucracy that required patients to be hospitalized even for minor treatments. Opponents of President Clinton's attempted health care reform portrayed the VA as proof of what would inevitably happen if government got more deeply involved in health care. Though more comprehensive reform of the system did not happen, in 1994 President Clinton did appoint Dr. Kenneth Kizer, MD, MPH, to head the VHA and re-engineer it into a top quality patient-centered, value-based system.

By 1998, Dr. Zizer's reform work had given him star status among managers. He had infused a commitment to continuous improvement into the "corporate culture" of the VHA. The bureaucracy was streamlined and reorganized on a practical level around the needs of the patients. A state-of-the-art computerized records system was developed and implemented to cover not only patient records but also to facilitate research on what interventions produced the best outcomes, allowing practices to be upgraded over the years. Seeking to control costs and aware that these veterans are clients for the rest of their lives, the VA sharpened its focus on primary care and prevention. Since its staff is all salaried, they have no incentive to either overtreat or undertreat. In his book *Best Care Anywhere*, Phillip Longman summarizes the VHA's cost-effectiveness: "Between 1999 and 2003, the number of patients enrolled in the VHA system increased by 70 percent, yet funding (not adjusted for inflation) increased by only 41 percent. So the VHA has not only become the health-care industry's best quality performer, it has done so while spending less and less on each patient."

The VHA has received many kinds of recognition for its outstanding quality of care. To list only a few examples, in 2003, the *New England Journal of Medicine* published a study comparing the VHA with fee-for-service Medicare on 11 measures of quality. The VHA was "significantly better" by all 11 measures. *The Annals of Internal Medicine* published another study revealing that the VHA topped major private managed-care systems on all seven metrics of diabetes treatment quality. A RAND study reported that the VHA outperformed all other sectors of American health care across a spectrum of 294 measures of quality in disease prevention and treatment. Harvard's Kennedy School of Government awarded the VHA its "Innovations in American Government" prize.

In his article "Health of Nations," Ezra Klein notes, "What makes this such an explosive story is that the VHA is a truly socialized medical system. The unquestioned leader in American health care is a government agency that employs 198,000 federal workers from five different unions, and nonetheless maintains short wait times and high consumer satisfaction. Eighty-three percent of VHA hospital patients say they are satisfied with their care, 69 percent report being seen within 20 minutes of scheduled appointments, and 93 percent see a specialist within 30 days."[10]

Increase the Supply of Medical Personnel

The Association of American Medical Colleges estimates that the United States will have a shortage of 63,000 primary care doctors by 2015, and the shortage will grow through 2025 unless strong corrective measures are taken now. A lengthy section of the law, known as Title V, deals in detail with expanding the number of providers among the many subgroups of medical personnel who are in short supply. The language conveys a strong sense of urgency. A shortage of medical personnel could become a bottleneck that slows the entire reform. Additional health care providers will be needed to care for the 35 million persons without insurance who are to be added to the rolls. Of particular concern are personnel to serve the low income, minority and rural populations. Graduating medical doctors have disproportionately chosen specialties, surgery and other high pay areas of medicine, rather than general practice. Geographically, they also tend to congregate in communities of more affluent people. The law makes the case that without a comprehensive strategy these shortages will grow.

Skilled technicians and allied health professionals who graduate from accredited programs can help alleviate the shortage by taking on some of the more routine tasks now being done by MDs. Others may begin careers as home health aides and continue with additional training from time to time in a "Health Care Career Pathway." They follow an established sequence of academic study and on-the-job training that leads to more responsible job designations, perhaps lower than a registered nurse but with significant responsibilities. The new law reflects the realization that it is time to "think outside the box" to streamline career pathways and expand career opportunities in order to address the growing problem of the medical workforce shortage.

Section C under Title V deals with increasing the supply of medical professionals in understaffed areas. This program increases funding for the National Health Service Corps, created in 1972, that awards scholarships to medical professionals in exchange for their commitment to practice in underserved areas for a specific number of years. This new emphasis is already seeing striking results. Thanks to stimulus money and funds from the ACA, the number of doctors and nurses participating is at its highest level since the Corps was created. About 10,000 clinicians are in the program serving some 10.5 million patients. Since 2009 the program has awarded medical professionals nearly $900 million in scholarships in exchange for their commitment to practice in both rural and urban locations. The new health care law provided $290 million of that funding. Officials expect the program to have an effect beyond the period of required service because 80% of corps members now continue to serve in high-need areas after they have fulfilled their time commitments.

The ACA mandates a "Health Care Work Force Commission" at the national level to evaluate education and training programs for all positions, determine whether needs are being met, and identify barriers to success. 15 members have been appointed by the Comptroller General for terms of three years. They will meet quarterly. The composition of members is designed to provide a balance of recognized experts from various parts of the country, city and rural, lay and professional. The Commission will submit an annual report to the President and Congress and make recommendations for change. There is real urgency in this effort.

Better Health through Research

The Affordable Care Act is packed with specific new research programs, along with funds for ongoing research.

We improve our collective health when we discover the relative effectiveness of different treatment options and then embed the best practices into the system. We study medical devices and learn the circumstances under which they should and should not be used. Research is especially needed on new drugs over the years after initial approval. The research reveals how to achieve higher quality health outcomes at lower cost. We illustrate with an example.

The *Harvard Health Letter* of March 2011 reported research on the proper use of the Implantable Cardioverter Defibrillator (ICD). This device, including batteries, is the size of a small cell phone. It is implanted under the skin with wires that snake through an artery and connect to the heart. Its purpose is to sense irregular heart-beats and then stimulate the heart back into a healthy rhythm.

Each month about 10,000 Americans have ICDs implanted under their skin. The hospital procedure and the device cost around $35,000.

The FDA approved the first ICD in 1985. Medicare began covering the cost a year later. Usage has grown steadily since then. But there is a problem: in many instances ICDs are overused. Device makers, of course, have a vested interest in selling more products. They hire salespeople to visit doctors and advocate for the benefits. Surgeons who implant the devices are compensated generously and the procedure helps keep hospital beds in use. Yes, there are always border-line situations when it is a judgment call whether or not to do the implant.

Research has recently revealed, however, that persons with no history of heart problems prior to a first attack do better taking appropriate medication rather than having an ICD implanted. Two studies sought to determine when it is appropriate to get the ICD. One study in 1995 looked at data for elderly people and found that only a few older people benefitted. Another more recent study examined whether doctors are following the guidelines of the American College of Cardiology. The research project studied records of 111,707 patients who received ICD implants between 2006 and 2009 on a "preventive" basis. The results were reported in the *Journal of the American Medical Association*. 25,145 patients or 22.5% who got one of the devices during that time period did not meet the guidelines for needing an ICD. Researchers calculated that at least 100 deaths occurred in this group because physicians overused the ICD. The study concluded, "… there is overuse without benefit, possible harm, and rising costs." At $35,000 per implant, this adds up to a waste of $880,075,000 per year, along with related health costs. [11]

Defective ICD devices are also sold to an unsuspecting public. They often go undetected without federal oversight and research. In January 2011, Boston Scientific, for example, agreed to pay a fine of $296 million after pleading guilty to charges they knowingly sold defective ICDs.

We raise a red flag against federal requirements that are so rigid they fail to take individual needs into account. However, it is clear that federal regulators must serve as vigilant watchdogs. The average person suffering from a heart attack has little time or means to evaluate the benefits or liabilities of treatment options or specific medical devices. Even busy doctors who are treating patients all day are not in a position to do all of their own research. Objective research should establish the norms of best practice and then some designated agency must be responsible for distributing that information throughout the medical community. Use of updated best practice standards based on on-going research will substantially improve health outcomes for all Americans over time.

A Case Study in Applying Medical Research to Improve Health Outcomes

Dr. Harlan Krumholz[12] is a cardiologist and professor at the Yale School of Medicine and Director of Yale-New Haven Hospital's Center for Outcome Research and Evaluation (COTE). He has devoted much of his research career to diagnosing what works and what doesn't for the American health care system. He directs graduate MDs at Yale as they learn how to produce better medical outcomes.

Dr. Krumholz has directed many blockbuster national studies, perhaps none more important than his campaign to lower the time between when a person has a heart attack and when the hospital performs angioplasty, a procedure that clears blocked arteries using a catheter and a balloon. Since the mid 1990s doctors knew that the chance for survival increased dramatically if the procedure could be done within 90 minutes of the time the patient arrived at the hospital. In 1995 the average time from "door to balloon" was about two hours. Most every hospital and cardiologist thought it was almost impossible to get below 90 minutes. But then Dr. Krumholz and his associates at Yale found that a few hospitals were achieving an hour and a half and even a shorter time. He and a team contacted the top performers to plumb their secrets. One key strategy was to let ER personnel diagnose a heart attack rather than wait for a cardiologist. They published a paper in the *New England Journal of Medicine* in 2006 detailing the ways they found to cut down on the time.

Dr. Krumholz was not satisfied with publishing a scientific finding; he wanted to translate it into national hospital practice. He launched in 2006 the D2B Alliance, a national campaign to reduce door-to-balloon time. Within its first year, the alliance enrolled 1,000 of the 1,400 hospitals that perform angioplasty, and in 2008 it met its national goal: 90 minutes from door to balloon for 75% of patients at the participating hospitals. The Alliance continued to expand and now Dr. Krumholz reports that many hospitals are beginning the procedure within 30 minutes. This represents a huge number of lives saved. He looks at problems of medical quality as "opportunities for improvement—focusing on solutions and progress."

This work inspired those who wrote the Affordable Care Act to create a nonprofit organization called the Patient-Centered Outcomes Research Institute (PCORI). It will conduct ongoing research on what treatments work best and how to spread information on best practices across the nation. PCORI will award more than three billion research dollars in the next decade. Dr. Krumholz is a leading member of the group's board of governors and will play a role in deciding where and how to spend that money.

Prevention Strategy Research, Ages 55 to 64

One research model in the Medicare section of the ACA is titled, "Healthy Aging, Living Well." The purpose is to provide evaluation of Medicare Community Based Prevention and Wellness Programs.

This Section provides $50,000,000 for pilot programs to implement prevention strategies in the age 55 to 64 population and research their effectiveness. This age group, the decade before Medicare enrollment, is important because many chronic illnesses begin during this period of life. Overweight during this decade leads to diabetes in later life. A sedentary lifestyle that begins at the television set in the late 50s leads to heart problems later. Quality of life, as reflected in better health, can be improved dramatically through such focused initiatives. The "hands-off" passive public attitude so prevalent now is leading to alarming increases in obesity, preventable chronic disease and higher health costs for Medicare.

The aim is to design strategies to promote healthy living and then evaluate the results in various geographical areas. Research grants are being awarded to communities through state and local health departments and on Indian Reservations. The focus is on improving nutrition, increasing physical exercise, improving mental health, reducing tobacco and substance abuse, etc. The projects will also study community effectiveness in helping persons enroll in appropriate insurance programs and find personal physicians in community networks. The demonstration begins by compiling baseline health data and then tracks health outcomes for that group over time.

Each research center that is awarded a grant keeps detailed electronic records and reports results to the Secretary of Health and Human Services. Research results from all of the pilot programs are then compared and further analyzed at the national level. A report will be sent to Congress, the President and relevant agencies. All data will be posted on the internet, available to consumers and providers. Ongoing community-based primary-care medical practice will be modified to reflect lessons learned from the research.

Overcoming Racial and Economic Disparities

We fall far short of attaining a healthy nation unless racial minorities and low income Americans have equal access to quality health care. Their quality of care now is demonstrably inferior. Add a backlog of "deferred maintenance" and we are faced with nothing less than a dismal swamp of festering health problems. For example, the infant mortality rate for African-Americans is twice that for non-Hispanic white Americans. The diabetes rate is almost double. And the list of such discrepancies goes on and on.

The National Cancer Institute statistics reveal that African American women die of cervical cancer at a rate of 4.4 per 100,000, while white women die at the rate of 2.2 per 100,000. The Institute cites disparity of access to health insurance as the primary cause. Leaders suggest that socio-economic factors could be mostly overcome by providing health insurance to everyone, in combination with an aggressive information and outreach program.

Care and compassion are evidenced throughout the 1000+ pages of the ACA. Special programs target these vulnerable populations, seeking to help break cycles of poor health from one generation to the next. Two examples provide a flavor of programs designed to improve health.

The law provides funds to states for grants to institutions of higher education to assist underserved females who are pregnant or have young children. These students will have help with maternity costs, child care, and commuting to class. The new mothers will attend classes to improve parenting skills, while medical services help get the new-born off to a healthy start. Funds are also available for counseling and referral services for adoption or foster care. Society is well-served when mother and baby have their health needs met, while the mother is getting a college education. This approach seeks to break the cycle of poor health, obstacles to education, and the despair of poverty for young single mothers.

Public school-based Health Centers are being established. Grants are available to public schools in areas where children are poor and health care is inadequate. Each school-based center will serve a high percentage of Medicaid children and adolescents. One section of the Act provides grants to prepare facilities in existing school buildings or on school grounds. A companion program provides funding annually for physicians, nurses, dentists, mental health professionals and others. The staff will provide in-school care and outpatient referrals. The Centers are designed to provide services during school hours, plus 24 hour "on call" service by backup providers. Centers will operate all 12 months of the year.

Many parts of the health care reform package are aimed specifically at helping low-income people, including 16 million new enrollees for Medicaid. This population has a significant portion of functionally illiterate persons. A study commissioned by the Institute of Medicine "Health Literacy Implications of the Affordable Care Act," released in November 2010, notes that 36% of American adults are functionally illiterate. Only 12% of adults have proficient health literacy, meaning they can readily understand health information and use it effectively. Health literacy does matter. Where it is lacking, the case manager or other non-physician must help interpret medical directives and see that they are carried out. This recognition is hugely important in providing better quality of health care for this population.

Quality of Care Must be Focused Locally

The best way to measure overall health is by studying longevity rates. A revealing study covering the years 1987 to 2007 was done by Christopher Murray and Sandeep Kuliarni of the Institute of Health Metrics and Evaluation at the University of Washington.[13] The study divided the nation into 2,400 units, most of which were counties or cities. It found that while average life expectancy has been gradually rising, in some areas children born now can expect to die sooner than their parents. In fact, in one quarter of the country, a girl born in 2011 can expect a life shorter than her mother's. The report found, further, that the country as a whole is falling farther behind other industrialized nations in the march toward longer life.

The study found that the extremes of good and poor health are often found within the same state. For example, in 2007 Fairfax County, Virginia had the longest life expectancy for men at 81.1 years. In the city of Petersburg, Virginia, 25 miles south of Richmond, life expectancy for men is 14 years less at 66.9 years, among the lowest in the nation. On an encouraging note, life expectancy can increase significantly over a ten year span. The District of Columbia had a life expectancy for African American men of 61.7 years in 1997. It jumped to 68.9 in 2007, a huge demographic improvement. This improvement, it must be acknowledged, was due in large part to the curbing of a crack cocaine epidemic.

Women lived longest in Naples and Collier County, Florida, at 86 years. Life expectancy is lowest in Holmes County, Mississippi at 73.5 years. Again, this is a 12.5 year spread in how long women typically live in different places. The region where life expectancy is lowest and is still declining begins in West Virginia, runs through southern Appalachia and west through the deep south into north Texas. Mississippi fares the worst among the states. The most striking trend in the study was the lower life expectancy for women. From 1997 to 2007 there were 860 cities or counties out of 2400 in which life expectancy for women decreased or stayed the same. For the first time in our history, the ACA appropriately emphasizes women's health issues.

The Affordable Care Act has the mission of concentrating resources and services in these low performing areas. Yet these are precisely the places where the state or local "establishment" most often resists plans to improve quality and coverage.

Protecting Health through Prevention

Beginning on September 23, 2013, new health insurance policies require insurers to provide a list of preventive procedures that must be delivered with no out-of-pocket cost to policyholders. These procedures include immunizations, cholesterol checks, colorectal cancer screening for people over 50, HIV screening for all adults in high-risk groups, depression screening for adults, obesity screening and counseling for adults, and tobacco screening for adults along with intervention for tobacco users. All women will have screening for breast cancer and be given birth control services with no co-payment. We will look in closer detail at several of these areas, beginning with immunizations.

Immunizing all Citizens

The Affordable Care Act grants authority to provide the public with all recommended vaccines free of charge. The Secretary of HHS is empowered to negotiate contracts with vaccine manufacturers for lowest prices to cover persons who receive service through federal programs. States may purchase amounts as needed under the same contracts. Funds are included to provide education and reminders to targeted populations. In places where few persons are immunized, public health nurses will be disbursed to promote and provide the service. Regular assessments will analyze the effectiveness of outreach. The goal is to remove barriers to immunization for the entire population as a public health safety precaution.

There is concern in the alternative medical community that immunizations may be overused and inadequately researched both before and after FDA approval. Some vaccines are contaminated with mercury and other harmful ingredients. Drug companies lobby heavily for new vaccines that are later shown to have questionable value, although they can be "cash cows" for the makers. Some question whether new-born babies should receive so many shots when there is little research on cumulative effects on immature immune systems. More careful independent research and oversight are necessary if life-saving vaccinations do not turn into death-producing nightmares.

Protecting Health through Annual Checkups

The ACA requires that every private health insurance policy and every government health program provide an annual checkup without co-pay to every enrollee. These exams offer an incredible opportunity to detect and address incipient health concerns before they become ravaging illnesses.

A recent research study sponsored by the National Institutes of Health revealed the benefits of such exams. The research staff analyzed data from 2008 for more than 14,000 men and women between ages 24 and 32. The survey looked specifically at high blood pressure among these young adults. There were two startling findings: (1) 19% of those in this study had high blood pressure, defined as a reading of 140/90 or higher and (2) only half of those with high blood pressure knew it. This study counters the oft repeated claim that young adults are healthy and do not need to see a doctor or get insurance. Second, it indicates a huge jump in high blood pressure among this age group, as the previous national estimate put the number at 4%. Finally, it says these young adults need to be under the vigilant care of a doctor so they can change their lifestyles, eat properly and get needed medication. It is tragic to contemplate heart attacks and strokes for persons in this age range.

Contraceptives among Preventive Services

The Affordable Care Act left it to the Department of Health and Human Services to determine what additional services should be required as part of a basic prevention package, based on recommendations from the National Institute of Medicine. During the first week of August 2011 the Obama administration announced they would accept the HHS recommendation that all FDA-approved contraceptives be included. The plan excludes employees of religious organizations that oppose contraceptive use but covers auxiliary organizations such as universities or hospitals that employ citizens from the general workforce who are not members of that faith. After an outcry from the Roman Catholic Church and others about interference with religious rights of conscience, the Obama White House found a compromise that allowed the Church to avoid paying for contraception while still allowing women to receive the services. Insurance Companies will pick up the tab, as contraceptive services are far less expensive than unwanted child births.

Nearly half of all pregnancies are unplanned, according to the Guttmacher Institute, and about 40% of women who find themselves with an unwanted pregnancy opt for abortion. Encouraging and underwriting contraception use reduces the number of abortions. Nine out of ten employer-based insurance policies already include this provision and 28 states have passed laws requiring insurers that cover prescription drugs to cover contraceptives. Providing contraceptive services to poor women is expected to improve the quality of life for them, with healthier children as an added bonus. The unintended pregnancy rate among poor women ages 15 to 44 rose from 88 per 1,000 women in 1994 to 132 per 1,000 women in 2006—a 50% increase. Over the same period, the rate among higher-income women in the same age group dropped from 34 to 24 per 1,000 women. **The pregnancy rate among poor women is about five times higher than that of higher-income women. The nation has an impending health crisis along with huge cost commitments unless this trend is reversed.**

The Guttmacher Institute also notes that unintended childbearing is often "associated with a number of adverse maternal behaviors and child health outcomes, including inadequate or delayed initiation of prenatal care, smoking and drinking during pregnancy, premature birth and lack of breast-feeding, as well as negative physical and mental health effects on children." The ACA declares that all women who are not financially or emotionally prepared for parenthood must have the same access to contraceptive services as the affluent now enjoy.

Other Special Programs for Women

The health care law directed the Obama administration to draw up a list of preventive and supportive services, in addition to contraceptive services, to meet the special needs of women. A commission has now made its recommendations, announced by HHS in July, 2011. If finally adopted, females will receive breast pump rentals, counseling for domestic violence and HIV tests, where appropriate.

Employers will be required to provide time for mothers to breast-feed their babies for one year after birth. A room must be made available other than a bathroom. If there are fewer than 50 employees and the policy would impose "undue hardship" the requirement may be waived. The provision invites states to pass laws requiring greater protection for mothers and babies.

Labeling Food to Improve Health

The ACA contains provisions to expand food labeling in an effort to raise nutrition awareness, encourage healthy eating and reverse the obesity epidemic. Chain restaurants with 20 or more locations must include nutritional information on the menus. Cafeterias must also display nutritional information about their foods. Grocery stores must expand the prominence and quality of labeling. The law even applies to food sold in vending machines. The Secretary shall also set "reasonable standards" for single- menu items such as soft drinks, ice cream, pizza, donuts, etc. Daily specials and temporary items are excluded.

There will be a concentrated public health effort to educate people on proper nutrition and give them the tools to make healthier choices.

Improving End of Life Care at Lower Cost

The Affordable Care Act supports a carefully constructed hospice system as an alternative to end of life in an intensive care hospital setting. The dying may choose to remain at home in a familiar setting surrounded by loved ones with support from hospice caregivers. For those not so fortunate as to have this option, hospice provides alternative home-like settings for the dying. Another option is palliative care in a more traditional hospital setting, following instructions from the patients to let them die without painful, intrusive and futile interventions.

Before a patient can be provided this type of care the person will have discussed the alternatives with family and decided that this is the most desired course. The person then writes a "living will," or advanced directive, that will have the force of a doctor's written order as a guide for care when a fatal illness comes. If a patient can no longer make wishes known and does not have an advanced directive, family can make this decision with a doctor concurring.

Patients often make these wills but they cannot be found at the crucial moment of a hospital crisis. Under the new law all records become electronic. The patient's primary care physician will note whether there is such a directive and have it on computer file before the crisis occurs. The decision can be to use every possible medical procedure, even in an unconscious state. Alternatively, the medical team and family, with the patient if possible, can decide the point where it is prudent to accept the fact of impending death, then manage pain and discomfort and let nature take its course. Whatever the statement dictates, it will become a permanent part of the medical records.

A team of physicians based at Oregon Health and Science University pioneered a one-page document called POLST (Physician Orders for Life-Sustaining Treatment). It is stored electronically and printed on the bed of the patient. The POLST program has proved so effective at getting patients the care they need in the way they want that the approach is now in use or is being developed in 30 other states and the District of Columbia. The model was used by those who designed the ACA. "Five Wishes," available through the Aging with Dignity website, is another very popular form of living will that also addresses emotional and spiritual desires of the individual.

The ACA allots funds to expand and improve the hospice system. Death can come with dignity and without unnecessary pain and suffering. Many families are finding hospice a far superior alternative. The cost is only a fraction of the highly expensive hospital end-of-life procedures and extended life-support. But again, the law gives the choice to the individual and is not, as many Republicans have charged, a way to "kill granny."

Summary and Conclusion

The programs outlined in this chapter offer an overview and illustrate provisions in the Act related to health care quality. A great deal of public money is spent not only to include virtually all of our citizens but also to improve the health of our population. Every member of society, rich and poor, benefits from many of these improvements, while the neglected and forgotten find themselves in a safe and caring nation for the first time.

We turn now to review and understand the many proposed savings included in the law.

Chapter 4

COST CONTROL

From 2000 to 2006 overall inflation increased 3.5%, wages increased 3.8%, and health care premiums increased 87%.

—Kaiser Family Foundation

The United States spends almost twice as much on health care per capita ($7,960) as any other country and spending continues to increase.

—Organization for Economic Cooperation and Development, 2009

Medicare operates with 3% overhead, non-profit insurance 16% overhead, and private (for profit) insurance 26% overhead.

—*Journal of American Medicine,* 2007

The health care system in today's America can be compared to the wild-west at the time settlers carved out homesteads and demanded law and order. The frontier included hunters, cattle thieves, cowboys, general store owners, saloon-keepers, bands of robbers and perhaps a few bankers. Each protected his own turf, and worked with others only when there was a direct benefit. A few got rich. Many more were gunned down and died. The six-gun was the law.

Eventually the west was tamed. Established norms of law replaced the six-gun. Towns sprang up for mutual support and well-being. States were formed. The cowboy gave up some freedom to gain the larger benefits of civil society. Settlers began to work for the common good.

With the Affordable Care Act comes a taming of our wild-west health care system.

We are hesitantly entering a new era of rational mutual benefit. But self-interested powerful robber barons still control much of the system. The general store owner who manages to charge twice what flour or shoes are worth has trouble adjusting to this new era. Those who love the free spirit of the old west are fighting hard to preserve their system of spoils. Yes, there are caring doctors who are in the profession because of their desire to serve. There are health insurance companies that follow the law and seek to provide the best service possible. But there are insufficient norms of good conduct and there are too many who yield to the temptation of making all of the money possible by insisting that laws favor them and by taking advantage of unregulated areas. And there are many who simply do not know best treatments or ways to become economically efficient. It all adds up. Other countries control their costs; we do not. Others achieve better health outcomes than we do. We can and must do better.

As late as the 1950s the doctors and the American Medical Association exercised control over medical practice and costs. Their primary concern was to maintain control over medical decisions while practicing as independent entrepreneurs. Their imaginations had not yet soared to the heights where they could envision practices based on large-scale profit centers with unending revenue growth.

Other big operators emerged. Much of the power shifted from the doctors to the health insurance companies after the defeat of health care legislation in the Clinton Administration. The insurance companies grew rapidly in size and wealth, and made billions in profits. Other corporate powers struck gold by buying the nation's hospitals. "Big Pharma" convinced Congress to give them stagecoach robbery profits for each new drug. The revised Medicare law in 2006 made it illegal for the government to negotiate drug prices, while pills were priced at up to a hundred times their cost. Medical device and equipment firms joined in reaping the spoils. Some surgeons, but also other specialists, began to charge thousands of dollars a day for their work. General practice doctors added "profit centers" to their practices.

America's health care system was evolving and each big player staked a claim to the abundant gold. As predictable as the rising of the sun or the presence of call girls above the old wild-west saloon, insurance rates rose annually as the many players found new veins of gold to mine. This gold, however, was being extracted from your pockets and mine. We were victims of powerful players and a mindless system. We were held hostage where we are most vulnerable—with our health. Yes, our lives!

Managing an Out-of-Control System

The Affordable Care Act is the first attempt to curb the greed and establish a system of law and order. It offers a best effort, under the political circumstances of our time, to establish a rational system of health care that reins in the avarice. For the first time in 60 years it proposes to put people first, ahead of profit. One of the three major goals of the Act is to find a way to control spiraling costs. As context for the need to control costs, the Act notes that "National health spending is projected to rise from $2,500 billion or 17.6% of the economy in 2009 to $4,700 billion in 2019." Cost saving is an effort to curb this huge increase. Out-of-control cost is not inevitable, but it will continue unless we stop it. We cannot stop it without establishing new "rules of the road." Those rules must be monitored. The Affordable Care Act has a chance to succeed because corporations, small businesses and individual citizens who are not wearing ideological blinders are all becoming painfully aware that the old system is out of control and unsustainable. Hence, many stakeholders are ready, with varying degrees of enthusiasm or resistance, to support fundamental changes to the system.

There is a world of savings to be mined. Huge bags of gold can be recovered by the once gullible public. Payday will come as we gain control over the avarice but also as we conserve the gold in a topsy-turvy mindless system where nobody thinks of saving. The Institute of Medicine estimated in October 2009 that a third of all health care spending in the United States—about $800 billion per year—goes to medical care that doesn't make us better.

When we examine health care systems in other countries we find three primary engines driving cost savings. First, governments purchase goods and services on behalf of individual citizens and drive hard bargains by purchasing in large lots. Government sees its role as saving money for the people. Even in Germany, where private health insurance plans compete with one another, they are not allowed to make a profit. Secondly, governments establish an annual national budget for health expenditures, taking into account the cost in prior years and making adjustments as necessary. Costs are then contained by paying only what the budget permits. Finally, governments use price regulation, as needed, to keep costs under control.

Legislators who wrote the Affordable Care Act were unable or unwilling to set such explicit standards for cost control. Clearly the law moves toward including each of these methods used in other countries, but in specific circumstances and situations rather than by sweeping design. The primary approach is to use a wide array of carrots and sticks rather than outright decrees. Each method of promoting savings can and should bring down costs over time, but each is subject to possible co-option by vested interests. The approach used in the legislation makes it difficult for the CBO and others to accurately predict the savings.

Restraining Growth of Insurance Premiums

Most of this chapter deals with restraining the growth of actual medical costs. Here we specifically address insurance costs. Of course, insurance companies must increase their premiums when their actual costs go up. Yet, an added concern is how to constrain the avarice of health insurance companies. The law does take steps to tame premiums. As indicated previously, it requires insurers to spend at least 80% of premiums on actual medical services, limiting their overhead and profit to 20%. It makes $250 million available to states for their staffs to analyze proposed rate increases to determine whether they are needed. It requires companies to justify their proposed increases and it requires them to fully disclose their costs and profits. The law also provides for federal review in states that are not equipped to do the job themselves. By mid-2011, the federal government had determined that 10 states won't be ready to adequately monitor companies' rate increases.

Kaiser Family Foundation did a national survey on the cost of insurance premiums for families in 2011. They found that the cost of family plan premiums for employer-sponsored health insurance escalated by nine percent in 2011. More bad news for employees: employers have moved to plans that require workers to pay more out of pocket. For the first time, half of workers at small firms with individual policies faced annual deductibles of $1,000 or more. At large firms, the share paid by the employee has grown from 6 percent to 22 percent in five years.

What explains this upward spiral? Americans continue to grow older. As citizens become poorer they lose insurance and therefore use the system less frequently in the short term, but accumulate larger health problems for the long term. The obesity epidemic is associated with increased economic stress. New diagnostic tools and procedures help drive costs. But the major culprit may be insurance companies' desire to raise premiums before controls and vigorous scrutiny kick in from the Affordable Care Act, beginning in 2012.

Critics say the new law is weak in that it leaves to each state the ultimate decision as to how much to permit rate increases. In mid 2011, 26 states had laws giving their state regulators authority to veto rates deemed excessive. Seven other states have the power to review rate increases in advance but not to block them. Other states without legal veto power are, on occasion, effective in negotiating with insurance companies. States that have funds to thoroughly analyze insurance company proposed increases have at times found important errors in the company calculations. For example, in 2010 Anthem BlueCross proposed a rate increase of 39% in California. Officials found and exposed glaring math errors, causing the company to withdraw the request.   The law demonstrates that it is crucial to make the rationale for an increase very transparent, so it can be checked. Much has been accomplished, but a state government that is in the pocket of the insurance industry can still do great harm to its citizens.[14]

Medical Spending versus Good Health

The Dartmouth Atlas hospital rankings and regional maps were used by the Obama Administration and the majority in Congress to deal with the lack of correlation between medical spending and the quality of patient care. Indeed, an article in the 2003 *Annals of Internal Medicine* states that "annual savings of up to 30% of Medicare expenditures could be achieved" by learning to use best practice strategies and by reigning in excessive costs, especially in some parts of the country. Dartmouth researchers now say that estimate was low. In recent interviews with *The New York Times* they stated that savings "substantially above 30 percent" were probable.

In too many instances health care costs and health care outcomes are not related. Why? It has become commonplace for most doctors, hospitals and other providers in some parts of the country to inflate their prices. Many doctors do what their colleagues do in a given community with the result that prices go up throughout the area. In addition, doctors in the same local medical society too often prescribe tests, treatments and surgery that are unnecessary and even injurious for the patient. They may justify the excesses by the need to protect themselves from malpractice suits. They may have a sense that, since the procedure exists, it should be used in the interest of thoroughness, even though the benefits may be marginal at best for the patient. Doctors often reinforce each other when ordering too many procedures that are counterproductive for patients, but highly lucrative for them. Yes, we live by habit, and over the years the habit of testing and over-treating patients who can pay has become commonplace. It is a sad truth that for some profit has become more important than providing good health care at the lowest price. When some players develop lucrative ways to successfully milk the system, their methods spread to friends and associates and the earlier service-oriented cultural values of the profession are corrupted by greed. The Act seeks to consciously lower costs in these inflated, high priced areas of the country.

Paying for the Affordable Care Law

First, it costs a lot of money to put this plan into place. More than 32 million new enrollees will get health care. That is expensive. Dozens of research projects are mandated to find cost efficiencies and best medical practices. The government offers tens of billions of dollars as incentives for players to switch to electronic records. Cost controls are mandated, requiring a new level of oversight for each of the big players. In summary, there is a negative cost associated with the Act. The Congressional Budget Office on March 30, 2011, issued a report estimating that health reform as envisioned will cost the U. S. Treasury $1.4 trillion from 2012 through 2021. This is an upward revision over the estimate made February 18, 2011 that projected a cost of $930 billion over that ten year period.

Part of this cost is recouped in the Act. It contains "offsets," built-in policies that offset the cost of the law. Some offsets are taxes while others are cuts in the cost of programs that are patently over-priced by providers. All are designed to help cover the costs. Here are examples of taxes and fees that are levied:

- Some high salaried corporate employees receive "golden" insurance policies from their companies as part of compensation packages. Their plans will be compared with the best "platinum" plan offered in their exchange. The employer pays a tax of 40% on all excess benefits. This tax is expected to raise $140 billion over ten years.
- Health insurance providers pay an annual fee based on net premiums written during a calendar year. Firms that do less than $25 million have the fee waived. Those whose business is in the range of $25 to $50 million pay half of the rate. Large firms doing annual business of more than $50 million pay the full amount. Foreign companies are included. The government expects these fees to raise $60 billion this decade.

- An excise tax of 3.2% is charged to medical device manufacturers and importers. This tax applies when the device sells for more than $100. It will raise some $13 billion over ten years.
- Similarly, there is a fee charged to large pharmaceutical companies that do significant business with the federal government. These fees should raise $27 billion this decade.
- In the Medicare part of the ACA an annual increase of .09% is levied on wages of individuals making more than $200,000 and couples making more than $250,000. In addition, these persons pay a 3.8% tax on unearned income including interest, dividends and capital gains. The amount increases to 5.4% on individuals making more than $1,000,000 per year on the part above $250,000. This money goes into a Hospital Trust Fund to help cover the costs of hospital care for the elderly. The Medicare tax is expected to raise $210 billion between 2013 and 2019.
- The Act limits to $500,000 the amount insurance companies can claim as a tax deduction for executive compensation.

"It takes money to make money." It costs money to get the new system in place and cover the costs of an expanding elderly population, mitigated by fees collected. But the savings outweigh the cost as we move down the road.

Savings often come through spending. For example, it costs money to crack down on "waste, fraud and abuse." Politicians when running for office sometimes claim they will balance the budget by routing out the crooks. This approach will not cure all fiscal ills, but it can help. There is known fraud in the Medicare and Medicaid systems of at least a billion dollars per year that can be detected and eliminated with enhanced enforcement capabilities. Of course, there has always been a unit in the Medicare law for dealing with fraud. But the new law adds far more money and develops new programs for law enforcement.

Criminals "work the system" by selling legitimate medical devices such as wheel chairs to elderly persons who do not need them. A doctor signs a request for funds to provide an enrollee with a motorized wheel chair. These ingenious devices can liberate immobile persons capable of using them. But there is fraud and abuse when the doctor conspires with the salesman to share the sale profits and authorizes 100 units instead of ten that are needed by his practice.

Another scheme, among many, is to sell a fraudulent device. The thieves steal a large number of names and social security numbers of older people. Someone signs the name of a legitimate physician. They provide an address for the company that turns out to be just a mailbox in a rundown building. Medicare is billed for a device that is non-existent or useless and the thieves collect.

The new law provides funds to root out such abusers. Additional enforcement personnel are being hired to investigate suspicious claims. New investigators are already at work under this law, beginning in large cities where government officials know there is significant abuse. Other methods of surveillance are being tried as pilot projects. One approach is to commission "Recovery Audit Contractors." These are individuals and small firms who specialize in following leads and uncovering overpayment. They work within prescribed limits and receive compensation based on the amount of money they recover.

On September 8, 2011 the Obama Administration announced the arrest of 91 persons in eight cities. They were accused of bilking Medicare out of nearly $300 million. For example, a doctor in Detroit allegedly billed Medicare for services provided to dead people and claimed he performed psychotherapy treatments more than 24 hours a day. The arrests, announced by Attorney General Eric H. Holder Jr. and Health and Human Services Secretary Kathleen Sebelius, marked another step in their campaign against fraud, a key part of the health care reform agenda. Altogether in 2011, the Departments of Justice and HHS recovered $4.1 billion in funds that had been stolen or improperly taken from federal programs. This was the highest amount for any year on record until that time. **A stronger, more effective Medicare Fraud Strike Force is now in place!**[15]

Savings from Universal Coverage

The Affordable Care Act had a series of amendments added at the end of the process that became part of the final law. In justifying the mandate that everyone have insurance, the law provides some basic statistics on cost savings from universal coverage. The economy loses up to $207 billion a year because of the poor health and shorter lifespan of the uninsured. Most of us have no idea of this drain on our economy. Consider three additional cost savings from universal coverage:

1. The cost of providing uncompensated care to the uninsured was $43 billion in 2008. To pay this cost hospitals passed it on to the insurance companies who, in turn, passed it on to families in the form of higher insurance premiums. The cost shifting increases family premiums by an average of $1,000 each year.

2. 62% of all bankruptcies are caused in part by costly medical expenses. Families are wiped out without enough insurance. Destitute families cannot pay physicians and hospitals for additional care.

3. Administrative costs for private health insurance, $90 billion in 2006, are 26% to 30% of premiums in the individual and small group markets. Overhead costs including profits are capped at 15% to 20% in the new law. A 10% reduction in these costs to the public amounts to $9 billion per year. Insurance companies agreed with President Obama to limit profits in exchange for obtaining 32 million new customers under ACA.

Patient-Centered Care Saves Money

Strangely, doctors in training have not been taught to focus on their patients. Medical schools teach a great deal of science but they devote little time to how one listens and learns during a patient visit. They take few, if any, courses on interpersonal relationships or even clinical judgment. Their role models are busy doctors in private practices, going as quickly as possible from one patient to another. The Affordable Care Act is determined to modify medical training to emphasize patient-centered care, to focus on improving health as much as treating illness.

They will be expected to listen more and get to know their patients over a period of years.

Doctors are challenged to use the best but simplest treatments. They are challenged to engage their clients in a practice that is person-centered, effective and relatively frugal. This is the new culture the ACA seeks to create. This approach has been demonstrated to improve patient health, if not doctors' profits.

Hospitals Have a Responsibility

The Affordable Care Act notes that hospitals are often inefficient and unhealthy, with unacceptable levels of hospital acquired infections and overcharges. It challenges hospitals to clean up and lower costs. The Act states, "Each hospital operating within the United States shall for each year...make public...a list of the hospital's charges for items and services provided." These hospitals will also be required to publish information related to protecting the health of patients and the rate of readmission of patients soon after release.

In each region of the country the Act establishes a "Medical Reimbursement Data Center" that deals with hospitals and other providers in that area. Its purpose is to collect data for the region and "develop fee schedules and other data-based rates...." The Affordable Care Act envisions moving toward standard fees that fairly and accurately reflect market rates. The data centers will update this information annually. This information will be used, in part, to constrain hospital billing.

How will this Data Center be useful? For one thing, it will monitor medical procedures to determine whether they are being used properly. For example, some hospitals overuse double CT scans.[16] Hundreds of hospitals routinely perform double scans as a type of chest imaging. Experts say the double scan should be used rarely, as it subjects patients to double doses of radiation, drives up the cost and is unnecessary for accurate results. In this test two scans are done at the same time, one using dye injected into the veins and the other without. A single scan with dye is adequate in virtually all circumstances, and in many cases the doctor does not even need dye, according to experts in the field. Yet some doctors believe there may be a slight edge in doing the double scan.

Nationwide in 2008 there were 76,781 double scans on Medicare patients, only 5.4% of total scans done. Yet 94 hospitals performed double scans on at least half their scan patients. The highest rate in the nation was at Memorial Medical Center of West Michigan that ran 89% of Medicare patients through the double scan. The Medical Reimbursement Data Centers are formed to monitor such practices and call their overuse into question.

Hospitals that use more double scans make more money. The double scan cost for a Medicare patient is $403, compared to $362 for a scan with single dye, and $245 for one without any dye. It is important to note also that patients who paid their own bills got the double scan for $284, a single scan with dye for $191, and one without dye for $153. Is Medicare being over-charged? Rosemary Gibson, co-author of "The Treatment Trap" and editor of a series of articles on overtreatment in the *Archives of Internal Medicine* commented, "This is one of thousands of things we do every day in health care that causes more harm than good. In addition to lowering quality of care, the overuse of double CT scans costs millions of dollars annually in overcharge."

Now we study other examples from the long list of savings embedded in the law.

Physicians' Abuse of their own Profit Centers

An interesting development is occurring in the medical delivery world. Practicing physicians look for ways to invest some of the money they are making. A group of doctors pool their resources and buy or build their own hospital or specialty medical center. These doctors then send their patients to their own hospitals or centers to use services on which they make a profit. Clearly, there is opportunity for conflict of interest and overuse.

Meanwhile, the U.S. Government Accounting Office (GAO) is investigating the practice. An official stated, "We need to figure out what's best for patients, not the bank accounts of urologists and radiation oncologists." The ACA is in the early stages of issuing regulations on this common practice, but the new law does permit doctors to refer their patients to their own facilities under limited circumstances.

The system is also being exploited by doctors who unite to purchase expensive diagnostic equipment. An article in *The Washington Post* reported on skyrocketing health costs because of this trend.[17] The article concluded, "Every ear, nose and throat doctor seems to have a CT scan machine. It is a huge driver of over-utilization." A Georgetown University health economist, Jean M. Mitchell, did a study showing that urologists who perform and receive payment for their own pathology services are more likely to order biopsies and take more tissue samples for analysis than those who don't.

Similarly, hospitals buy extremely expensive new equipment and then overuse it in order to recoup the cost. For example, robotic surgery is "the new kid on the block." It is being advertised as the next great leap forward in medical technology. Surgeons sit and watch a video console that displays three-dimensional images. They use computer controls to guide the robotic arms that maneuver the surgical instruments inside the body. The robot and the computer software cost in excess of a million dollars. In addition, each operation uses disposable robots that are replaced in the next operation.

Dr. Richard Hodin, MD, of Massachusetts General Hospital comments, "It is impressive technology, but what are the benefits? Unfortunately, up to this point, there's remarkably little, if any, evidence that robotic surgery helps the patient or the surgeon…. Yet more hospitals are buying these machines, not out of any real medical need or demonstrated advantage, but because of smart, skillful marketing by the companies that make them. Once a hospital has robotic surgery equipment, it needs to justify the cost by marketing it to the public."[18]

Ending Overpayment to Medicare Advantage

A major unnecessary cost that the Affordable Care Act addresses is overpayment in the Medicare Advantage program. The "Medicare Advantage" law was pushed through the Senate in the middle of the night in 2006 by a Republican Congress. This scheme requires the government to subsidize private insurance for Medicare recipients, adding billions of dollars each year to the cost. The Advantage program is voluntary and seniors pay on average $39 per month to belong. Doctors like the plan because they are paid more. Private insurance companies like the plan because they get paid at a higher rate. Under ACA, terms of the Medicare Advantage Program are revised gradually to make Medicare reduce the inequities and lower costs by billions of dollars.

The Medicare Payment Advisory Commission (MedPAC) estimates (2010 study) that Medicare paid these plans 14% or $1,000 per person more for health services than they did for traditional Medicare recipients, with no measurable difference in health outcomes. Ultimately, these overpayments cost all Medicare recipients additional funds, including the 75% who are not enrolled in the Advantage program.[19]

Ending Overpayment for Medicare Part D

When Medicare Part D was passed to include drug coverage for seniors, Republicans insisted that the government be barred from negotiating better prices with the pharmaceutical companies for billions of dollars worth of drugs. This was a massive bonanza for the pharmaceutical companies because the government had to pay exorbitant retail prices. Yes, Uncle Sam negotiates in the Veterans Health Administration to control costs there, but not in Medicare. This golden bonanza for drug manufacturers was a financial disaster for Uncle Sam and millions of seniors on Medicare who pay 20% of the cost from their own accounts.   Under the new law government will, in fact, save billions of dollars by negotiating best prices for Medicare. We now consider other ways to save on pharmaceutical costs.

Controlling the Cost of Prescription Drugs

The law recognizes that billions of dollars can be saved annually by reducing medication costs. Most of us are familiar with generic drugs, chemically identical to the original expensive versions, that are usually sold for pennies on the dollar. Yet doctors often fail to request the lower-cost generic drugs. A study conducted by Consumer Reports National Research Center[20] states that just 5% of patients learn about the price of prescribed drugs during doctor visits. For example, doctors routinely prescribe Nexium for acid reflux, costing $248 per month. However, an over-the-counter alternative, Prilosec, works the same way and costs only $24 per month. Physicians prescribe Lovaza for high triglycerides at $213 per month. As an alternative, fish-oil capsules cost $10 per month. The list of unnecessarily expensive prescriptions goes on indefinitely. The ACA adds controls and oversight that should greatly limit this wasteful practice.

The question remains as to how the law will treat soaring, even outrageous, pricing when only a single effective drug is available, or when a break-through drug is new on the market. Two examples will illustrate the dilemma. First, the FDA approved a compound called Makena, composed of two older drugs no longer widely used that were found to prevent premature birth when combined. Doctors and prospective parents cheered until they saw the price tag. KV Pharmaceutical of St. Louis sells Makena for $1,500 per dose and it must be injected every week for 20 weeks, at a cost of $30,000 per pregnancy. The two older drug components of Makena used to be sold for $10 to $20 each before researchers realized the value of combining them. There are more than 500,000 women each year who give birth prematurely out of a total of 4.2 million babies born. If the price is permitted to remain, it will swell the total cost for these high-risk pregnancies by more than $4 billion annually. Critics note that the approval process cost just $5 million and was paid by taxpayers. The approval gave Makena seven years of exclusive rights to sell the drug. The FDA said they had no idea how much the company planned to charge.

Other companies, emboldened by the ACA, have recently started producing a cheap version of Makena, in violation of KV Pharmaceutical's exclusive rights. In a statement released on March 30, 2011 the FDA announced that the "FDA does not intend to take enforcement action against pharmacies that compound the agent." The Agency was supported by Members of Congress who made their views known. KV Pharmaceutical said they take seriously the criticism of their pricing and will announce solutions soon. This company previously would have made billions of dollars from this drug. Their profits will be limited now to a reasonable amount, due to pressure from the new Affordable Care Act.

A second example is the struggle within the Medicare organization over whether to approve payment for Provenge as a cancer drug. This new drug is used for treatment of prostate cancer at a cost of $93,000 per patient. The Centers for Medicare and Medicaid Services (CMS) at first proposed to pay for Provenge stating, "The evidence is adequate to conclude that Provenge improves health outcomes for Medicare beneficiaries and thus is reasonable and necessary." CMS decided, however, to launch a formal investigation after passage of the ACA. Doctors use this drug when the prostate cancer is in an advanced stage. Researchers found that it extends the patient's life by four months on average. The campaign to win approval to pay for the drug has raged since 2007. Supporters of the drug have inundated CMS with hundreds of thousands of comments. Here is the moral dilemma: does the government spend $93,000 plus other medical costs to prolong the life of an elderly ill man for an additional four months? Is this, on the other hand, a reasonable place to "ration" medical care, given the need to cut overall costs?

Let the Computer Do the Saving

Full utilization of the computer is expected to save billions of dollars. The new law envisions consistent, rational computerized forms and records, to be used by all insurance companies and doctors. Medical offices now employ large staffs to prepare and submit complex insurance forms that are inconsistent from one insurance company to another. This expense will be reduced significantly, using electronic records and standardized claim forms. The new system will also reduce confusion for the patient who now receives multiple billings and requests for money. The U.S. Postal Service is the only group that will lose from an electronic system! Every government agency and every corporation in America uses computers to lower costs and improve quality. Can doctors and hospitals be far behind?

Cost Savings through Innovation

The "Independence At Home Demonstration" for the elderly is an innovative experiment sponsored by Medicare and Medicaid. The population to be served is the frail elderly and/or the chronically ill. When unable to be cared for at home, they now have no alternative but to move to a nursing home, an extremely costly placement that is often used only because Medicaid will not pay for a less expensive option. The demonstration tests a payment incentive and service model. A home-based primary care team agrees that for a specific amount of money for a year they will provide care to 200 persons or more in their homes. The care must be "comprehensive, continuous and accessible." The staff must be available for emergency care whenever it is needed. They agree to keep electronic records of all their services to each client. They agree to purchase a van with a mobile diagnostic center. They receive incentives for both savings and good health outcomes. The demonstration includes a program to reduce the wasteful dispensing of drugs, so common now in nursing homes. CBO analysts expect this type of reorganization to save the state and federal government billions of dollars annually. Nursing homes charge an average of $320 per day. Medicaid now spends half of its budget on nursing home care. Huge sums of money can be saved if people can be cared for less expensively at home. Most elderly people prefer to remain in their own homes if they can, so this alternative to nursing home care will be a win-win for all.

CBO Analysis of Preventive Services

We come now to cost control through preventive medical services such as cancer screening, cholesterol management, vaccines and birth control. The ACA also emphasizes wellness through smoking cession, obesity reduction, improved nutrition and encouragement of exercise. Legislators expected these measures to provide substantial savings. When the House Committee on Health, Energy and Commerce wrote to the Congressional Budget Office (CBO) asking them to score the savings, the reply was disappointing and ambiguous to the legislators.[21]

The CBO's response pointed out that different types of preventive care have differing costs and benefits. But generally, the savings are less than intuitive observation would suggest. A vaccination initiative, for example, might save the lives of a large number of persons. But the cost of administering it to a very large population might cancel the savings. The letter made it clear that the public policy decision to provide the vaccination could be made to save lives, whether or not it saved money.

The other major focus of the letter was the cost-effectiveness of wellness programs. First, smoking prevention will save significant money. Studies show that 10% of the total health bill for the nation could be eliminated if everyone were to give up tobacco. Obesity is recognized as the newest public health problem driving up costs, but the CBO has no way to evaluate now how much money will be saved through education, awareness programs, improved school lunches and the many other ways to control obesity. They conclude that we have to eat and there are many factors that affect our weight, making savings difficult to evaluate.

Two other considerations must be factored into whether there will be savings from wellness programs. First, the longer people live because of improved health, the more their health care may cost over a longer lifetime. Second, some people are already receiving some of the preventive services that will be provided for everyone in the Act. This will not increase total costs to society, but it may transfer some of the costs from individuals to the government.

The bottom line is that the CBO is unwilling to predict an amount that can be saved through prevention and wellness programs. Nonetheless, the legislators, the medical community and policy analysts continue to believe that the public mindset can and must be shifted toward staying healthy. They continue to believe this will result in significant health care savings. The scoring will have to come later.

With these caveats in mind, let us examine potential cost savings made possible by promoting wellness.

Smoking Cession

The Affordable Care Act deals with programs to reduce or stop smoking, long recognized as a major public health expense. The medical cost of smoking is enormous but, thankfully, tobacco use is going down. 1950 was a significant year for cigarette makers and users; the first major study was published showing the link between smoking and lung cancer. That year more than half the people in our country smoked. We were losing over 400,000 people a year to agonizing death from lung cancer.

Then the government began a concerted drive to educate the public and slow the use of tobacco. Statistics showed a decrease in cigarette use that coincided with periods of increased publicity concerning the health hazards of cigarette smoking. The first major thrust of published articles and news stories appeared in the popular press in 1953 and 1954, when there was a modest drop in smoking. The first report of the Advisory Committee to the Surgeon General appeared in January 1964. This was followed in July 1966 by the Federal Cigarette Labeling and Advertising Act, requiring a health warning in all advertising and on every package. By this time the percentage of smokers in the population had fallen to 41.7%. The Federal Communications Commission applied the Fairness Doctrine to cigarette advertising, ruling that broadcast stations carrying cigarette commercials must devote a significant amount of time to informing listeners of the health hazards of smoking. By 1978 the percentage of smokers had dropped to 33.2%.

States and local communities began to ban smoking in restaurants, bars, and on public transportation. Employers banned smoking in work places or they set aside rooms for smoking. The public became increasingly intolerant of secondary smoke. The percentage of smokers in 2007 had dropped to 19.8%, or 21.1% for men and 18.3% for women. **Over the past 60 years, the percentage of smokers in the population has fallen from more than 50% to less than 20%. This significant reduction demonstrates that a strong public information program can make an** enormous difference in public health outcomes and expenditures.

Cigarette manufacturers are now finding a way to again increase tobacco sales by advertising menthol cigarettes to minority youth. An FDA panel report of March 2011 stated that 80% of adolescent African American smokers use menthol cigarettes. Only slightly lower numbers were found among Hispanic American and Asian American youth who smoke. The FDA concluded that menthol was added because it eliminated the harshness experienced without it. The FDA also found that more than 90% of adult smokers became hooked on tobacco as teens. Lorillard and J.R. Reynolds tobacco companies have gone to court to block the FDA from considering the panel's recommendation to prohibit the use of menthol or other flavoring that makes cigarettes more attractive to teens. The Department of Health and Human Services responds that the new health care law has made a commitment to reducing health costs. Congress stated in the Tobacco Control Act that, **"Reducing the use of tobacco by minors by 50% would prevent well over 10 million of today's children from becoming regular, daily smokers. Such a reduction in youth smoking would also result in approximately $75 billion in annual savings attributable to reduced health care costs."**

These data led those who wrote the ACA to conclude that even further reductions in smoking are possible. They concluded further that eating healthy foods, weight management, exercise programs and other aspects of wellness can make major advances in keeping America healthy through public education and awareness efforts, as has the tobacco awareness program. Hence, a host of specific programs are detailed in the Act that promote public awareness, provide incentives for wellness and reduce costs.

Dealing with Obesity

The United States is in the midst of an obesity crisis. Over half the population is overweight and 25% are obese. The human and financial costs are almost unimaginable. The *Journal on Health Affairs* reported in 2009 that medical costs for those truly obese were $150 billion in 2008. Observers are concerned that one in three children has fallen into obesity or severe overweight. Data shows that obesity increased in 38 states and decreased in none during 2010. According to Dr. Ken Fujioka who directs the Nutrition and Metabolic Research Center at the Scripps Clinic in San Diego, "It is quite clear that once someone gains weight, the body will turn on a host of defense mechanisms to maintain that higher weight. Most people are trying to fight biology and not just habits when they try to lose weight."

Obesity has properly been called an "epidemic" because the percentage of obese adults has doubled in the past 40 years, and childhood obesity is increasing even more rapidly. According to a study quoted by the National Institutes of Health, "Obesity is associated with over 112,000 excess deaths due to cardiovascular disease, over 15,000 excess deaths due to cancer and 35,000 deaths due to a variety of other causes that would not have occurred if persons were of normal weight."[22] Health care costs for these obese persons are 42 percent higher than for persons whose weight falls into the normal range.

Medicare costs are $1,723 per year more for the obese beneficiary than the non-obese one.

The goal should be to prevent obesity in the first place. That is why first lady Michelle Obama has made childhood obesity her signature issue. In a speech last year to food manufacturers and retailers, the first lady urged them to stop marketing unhealthy foods. She said, "Our kids didn't learn about the latest sweets and snack foods on their own. They heard about these products from advertisements on TV, the Internet, video games, schools and many other places."

The Affordable Care Act calls for guidelines that limit advertising junk foods filled with sugar, salt and fat to children. "We allow companies into our homes to manipulate children to want food that will make them sick," said Margo Wootan of the Center for Science in the Public Interest, which is leading a coalition of public health groups to support the ACA's stringent guidelines on advertising food products to children. **The food industry spends about $2 billion each year marketing obesity-inducing products directly to children**.

Can Wellness Interventions Reduce Costs?

Though the Congressional Budget Office declines to calculate expected reductions in health care expenditures related to wellness interventions because of insufficient experience and research, we can still explore potentials in this direction.

In addition to interventions aimed specifically at smoking cessation and obesity control, other lifestyle interventions aim at stress reduction. In a study reported in the *American Journal of Health Promotion*, a group of researchers attempted to analyze the relative contributions of various lifestyle factors to medical expenses. They reported: "Stress was the most costly factor, with tobacco use, overweight, and lack of exercise also being linked to substantial expenditures."[23] Chronic stress is known to adversely affect several physiological systems and to contribute to a wide range of physical and mental disorders. Chronic stress also contributes to unhealthy lifestyle behaviors such as smoking and overeating.

Certain forms of meditation and relaxation techniques have been researched and found to cause significant health improvements. The best researched and perhaps the most effective[24] has been the Transcendental Meditation technique, a very specific but easy to learn technique that yields a wide array of documented positive effects ranging from reduced blood pressure to reduced anxiety to increased learning ability.[25]

Another extensively researched intervention[26] is taught by the Institute of HeartMath. The HeartMath group teaches simple techniques that improve heart rate variability, along with many related physiological benefits. Over time, practitioners can learn to function with more emotional intelligence and a more balanced physiology, using techniques taught by the Institute and a simple biofeedback device that allows the user to favor responses that produce the desired results.

Case Study: Teaching the Transcendental Meditation (TM) Technique to High-Cost Health Care Consumers.

This preliminary study, published in the *American Journal of Health Promotion,*[27] was conducted in Quebec, Canada, where the single-payer system makes it easy to track total physician expenditures for individuals.   It focused on the 10% of the people in the system who incurred the highest expenses.

In the U.S., the 10% of the general population that spends the most on health care accounts for 60-70% of total medical expenditures per year.[28][29][30]   In the Medicare population, the 5% that spends the most accounts for 40-45% of total Medicare expenditures.[31][32] The high-expense groups tend to have very poor health, usually suffering from several chronic health problems over a long period of time. The idea behind this study was that, if this difficult-to-treat group could be helped by a different type of intervention, significant cost-reducing leverage could be achieved for the system.

This retrospective study compared the highest-spending 10% of 1418 Quebec health insurance enrollees who practiced the TM technique with the highest 10% of 1418 matched control subjects who were randomly selected by RAMQ (Quebec's provincial government health insurance agency) from enrollees of the same age, sex, and region. Baseline physician expenses were taken from the year before the TM participants learned the technique, and physician expenses were tracked for both groups for the 5 years after the TM group started.

The TM group's physicians' expenses fell over the 5 year period with a statistically significant cumulative reduction of 28% of expenses on average. The control group's expenses fell only 2%, which was not statistically significant.

Although there is a large body of research on the effectiveness of stress-reduction interventions, research specifically focused on consequent reduction in medical expenses is minimal. We need more.

Specific Wellness Initiatives in the ACA

- Medical school curriculums and training programs for other health care providers will be updated to emphasize wellness and to promote it effectively.
- Employers will get financial incentives to provide physical training facilities for employees. Some employers already provide on-site gyms but this program will give more people easy access to gym workouts.
- Employees will receive reduced co-payments on their insurance or cash incentives when they stop smoking, lose weight and get regular checkups.
- Public schools will focus on healthier meals for students, offer health and nutrition education, and set aside more time for recess and physical education.
- Movie stars and popular athlete role models will be enlisted to promote healthy life-styles.
- Grocery stores will provide nutritional labeling of every food product sold, giving calories and complete nutritional information.

- Stress reduction classes and programs will be encouraged, as persons with high stress levels are shown to be more susceptible to disease and illness.
- Public health officials will work with urban governments to encourage elimination of "food deserts" in inner cities. These desert areas have no full-service grocery stores that sell fruits and fresh vegetables at reasonable prices, leaving inner-city residents without access to proper foods.
- Chain restaurants with more than 25 outlets, as well as cafeterias and vending machines that sell food, are required to post calories and nutritional information on the foods they sell.
- Public health officials will work with communities to encourage the creation of bicycle lanes and walking trails in neighborhoods.
- Public health officials will increase immunization initiatives to prevent outbreaks of infectious diseases. They will work more closely with pharmaceutical companies to develop new vaccines and will negotiate cost control.
- Every Community Health Center, every Accountable Care Organization, and every Medicare service provider will be asked to focus on wellness programs.
- Major research programs will evaluate results from specific initiatives so that wellness efforts can become more effective over time.

The Ultimate Weapon in Cost Control

The increasing cost of Medicare is a major cause of concern for the future. The baby-boomers are aging and are enrolling in Medicare, while at the same time health care costs per person are rising more than two percentage points per year faster than Gross Domestic Product (GDP). Cynics say these cost saving measures sound like good ideas on paper, but they probably won't produce the expected results. What if costs continue to rise much faster than one percentage point of GDP?

A crucial provision of the ACA is the creation of the Independent Payment Advisory Board (IPAB) to provide back-up cost control. This Board, due to begin functioning in 2013, is mandated to propose cuts in Medicare to Congress if spending grows by more than one percent faster than the gross domestic product. If Congress should fail to make these cuts, the Department of Health and Human Services is authorized to follow the recommendations of the Board and lower costs in ways it designates. It is a last resort, a fail-safe mechanism. Cost control must happen.

A great hue and cry has burst forth across the land as opponents claim "doomsday." Every special interest group that has a favored seat at the table due to hard lobbying of Congress fears its potential loss. **Those calling for major spending cuts throughout the government are the same persons seeking the destruction of the IPAB, whose primary task is to guarantee these savings!** The *National Review* was typical of ACA opponents when it described the IPAB as "the real death panel, the true seat of rationing, and the royal road to health care socialism."[33]

Cost Savings on Medicare

We have more accurate knowledge of costs and potential savings for Medicare than for other parts of the system because Medicare has a staff, employed over a long time period, to do actuarial studies that can predict savings. Many of the savings achieved in Medicare will be reflected in similar savings throughout the health care system.

First, there will be savings for individual Medicare participants. Seniors pay 20% of their costs out of pocket under Medicare part B. The Office of Planning and Evaluation in the U.S. Department of Health and Human Services projected the level of savings over ten years for individual Medicare recipients. The study estimates that seniors will save an average of $3,500 over ten years on their 20%. Those who take several expensive prescription drugs could have out-of-pocket savings as high as $12,500 over ten years.

Huge savings will come to the Medicare system. The Office of the Actuary at the Center for Medicare and Medicaid Services studied the effects of the ACA on Medicare costs. They concluded[34] that the Affordable Care Act "extends the life of the Medicare Hospital Insurance Trust Fund by 12 years, from 2017 to 2029." It adds $575 billion to the Trust Fund over the next ten years. Without the Act Medicare was projected to grow at an annual rate of 6.8%. As a result of the Act, growth is expected to be 5.3%, a saving of $575 billion over ten years.

Here is a listing of the specific major categories of savings that are projected by the Office of the Actuary:

Savings Type	10 Year Savings
Improved productivity of providers	$205 billion
End overpayment to Medicare Advantage	$145 billion
Independent Payment Advisory Board	$23.7 billion
Stop overuse of medical equipment	$17 billion
Reduce hospital readmissions	$8.2 billion
ACOs with revised payment structure	$4.9 billion
Waste, Fraud and Abuse reduction	$4.6 billion
Reduce hospital mistakes	$3.2 billion
Modify payments for advanced imaging	$2.0 billion
Improved physician reporting	$1.96 billion

Medicare, like Social Security, is a "pay as you go" system that depends primarily on today's working population to fund the expense of today's beneficiaries. For many years more money has been paid into the system than has been expended, in anticipation of the baby boomers reaching the eligibility age. Money not immediately paid out was invested in federal treasuries, loaned to the federal government to cover debt obligations. From the point of view of the Medicare Trust Fund, this has worked so far because there were many more workers than older people, but now that ratio is shifting. In 2010 there were 46 million seniors with 3.7 active workers per senior. In 2020 the number shifts to 61 million older persons and 2.9 workers per senior, while in 2030 the ratio shifts further to 78 million on Medicare with 2.4 workers paying into the system for every Medicare recipient. The problem is exacerbated further by the fact that medical costs throughout the system have risen an average of 2.5% faster than the general economy.

The ACA attempts to address the financial challenges specific to the demographics of Medicare as well as the financial challenges to the system as a whole. In 2011, for the first time, Medicare participants who are more affluent will pay a higher fee for services. In addition, about 1.2 million of the 28 million people who have Medicare prescription drug benefits must pay more for them. And the proportion of older Americans who pay higher premiums for coverage of doctor visits is expected to increase from 5% to 14% by the end of the decade. The Affordable Care Act required several new taxes on the more affluent, along with the other new efficiencies and savings.

Medicare is the most efficiently administered part of our health insurance system. Only 3% of every dollar spent goes for administration, whereas private health insurance companies have traditionally spent 25% or more for overhead, lavish salaries for top executives, and profits. One wonders why Republicans are working so hard to undermine Medicare when it gives us our best leverage for lowering costs.

Will Costs Be Controlled?

Cost control is the third leg of the tripod, one of the three purposes of the Affordable Care Act. As a society, we have little choice but to see this through to the end. How well the new law controls cost will be determined by how much influence each special interest group can garner in the halls of Congress, at state capitols, and with the regulatory agencies. That, in turn, is partly dependent on whether the Republican Party continues to represent special interests at the expense of the common good. The truth be told, most Republicans prefer cost control obtained by junking universal coverage, and letting the poor fend for themselves.

We can harness this beast over time and save our society if we have the public will to do so. This effort must include the IPAB to do cost analysis and control. We have staked our financial future as a society on being able to keep costs within bounds we can afford. While IPAB serves Medicare alone, supporters expect its decisions to influence cost control in the entire health system. Should that fail to happen, we will need a different version of IPAB to serve the remainder of our system.

Any observant person realizes that all cost predictions are estimates of what is perceived to be the most likely course of events. CBO claims authority because it makes projections based on past results and the terms of the law as written at the time the prediction is made. Much of the ACA is new, based on reasonable expectations and small successful experiments. It sets forth a process as much as a product. It emphasizes experimentation, careful recording of results and then sharing widely the things that are successful. But it also attempts to build on a solid foundation of managing our system as a whole for the benefit of the citizens—the common good. Many of us expect the cost savings to be far greater than projected, as we develop a new mind-set of staying healthy and as we judiciously use medical interventions with a keen eye on cost control.

Republican Congressman Paul Ryan, Budget Committee Chairman, presented his cost-cutting plan that changes Medicare from a guaranteed insurance program to a voucher program using private insurance and dramatically increasing the amount seniors would pay for services. When Democrats objected, Mr. Ryan said, "We have been bold. We have a plan to save Medicare. Democrats object to our plan, but they do not have one of their own."

Nancy Pelosi, former Democratic Speaker of the House, was asked to respond. She said, "Tell Mr. Ryan that we passed the Affordable Care Act!"

Chapter 5

HEALTH CARE IN OTHER COUNTRIES

The United States ranks 43rd in lowest infant mortality
rate, down from 12th in 1960 and 21st in 1990. Singapore
has the lowest rate with 2.3 deaths per 1000 live births,
while the United States has a rate of 6.3 deaths per 1000
live births.

—CIA Factbook, 2008

While numbers can be manipulated to make a
scoundrel seem honest, honest numbers, fairly presented,
don't lie. The numbers provided below by the
Organization for Economic Cooperation and Development
(OECD) reveal the quality of health in each country as
measured by life expectancy and infant mortality, along
with the cost per person, the percentage of government
revenue spent on health care and finally, the percentage of
health costs paid by the government.

COUNTRY	Life Expect -ancy	Infant Mortal -ity per 1000 Births	Per Capita Cost	Gov't Income toward Health Care	Health Costs Paid by Gov't
Germany	79.8	3.8	$3,588	17.6%	76.9%
France	81.0	4.0	$3,601	14.2%	79.0%
UK	79.1	4.8	$2,992	15.8%	81.7%
Japan	82.6	2.6	$2,581	16.8%	81.3%
Sweden	81.0	2.5	$3,323	13.6%	81.7%
Canada	80.7	5.0	$3,895	16.7%	69.8%
USA	78.9	6.7	$7,290	18.5%	45.4%

Source: http://www.oecd.org

Does it take your breath away, as it does mine, to learn that the United States is 42nd among nations in the rate of infant mortality, while also having a lower life expectancy?   Study the chart above and note that our country falls behind these other developed countries in every category.   Yes, our government contributes only 45.4% of the total cost of our health care yet we spend the highest percentage of our gross domestic product on health care at 18.5%.   We can count that a victory, if we are doctrinaire believers in free enterprise.   However, even opponents of the Affordable Care Act must concede that we pay a high price for an irrational, fragmented health care system.   **In fact, we pay almost twice as much per capita as these other systems and get inferior results**. Our high per capita cost is even more outrageous than it seems when you consider that this represents an average cost. The substantial portion of our population that lacks access to health care obviously does not spend much, yet these citizens are included in the average. So even more is actually spent on those who do receive care.

How do these other countries manage to include all their citizens while we are not able to do so? How do they manage to keep costs under control, while our costs run wild? How do they manage to achieve high quality, while our system falls behind, as evidenced by our being 42nd in infant mortality? Let's examine more closely the systems in these six countries most comparable to our own.

The Health Care System of Germany

Germany has the oldest health care system in Europe and one of the oldest in the world. Its origin was in The Health Insurance Bill of 1883, the Accident Insurance Bill of 1884 and the Old Age and Disability Insurance Bill of 1889. The insurance was mandatory but originally it applied only to low-income workers and government employees. It then gradually expanded into universal coverage. Today 99.8% of the population is covered.

German people pay into what is known as a "sickness fund." The government requires lower and middle income people to enroll in these sickness funds, but richer persons can opt out and choose their own private insurance plans. Currently, 83% of the population is covered by a basic health insurance plan provided by the state; the others opt for a private insurance company that includes all of the benefits of public insurance, often with additional benefits. Approximately 90% of German people take a private supplemental insurance policy to cover items not included under their standard insurance, much like American Medicare seniors can add a supplementary insurance policy. According to the World Health Organization, Germany's health system is about 77% government funded and 23% privately funded.

The government helps to pay the premiums of lower income citizens on a sliding scale. Similarly, higher wage earners pay insurance premiums based on their salaries. Co-payments were introduced in the 1980s in an attempt to limit utilization. Hospital reimbursement is based largely on the number of patient days rather than on the number of procedures. The sickness funds reimburse doctors on a fee-for-service basis, but fee amounts are controlled and the number of physicians in a given area is regulated by the government working in conjunction with professional medical societies.

German citizens are offered three policies: health insurance, accident insurance, and long-term care insurance, usually for old age. The health insurance cost is from 10% to 15% of the worker's salary, but half the cost is paid by the employer. Spouses and children are included free and other family members may be enrolled for a fee. The employer pays the total cost of accident insurance on the job, including insurance while traveling to and from work. The long-term care fund is paid jointly by employer and worker.

German health benefits are very generous for those in the system, including all illegal residents and visitors. There is usually no wait for elective surgery or diagnostic tests. Germans believe they have one of the best systems in the world and are overwhelmingly supportive of it. Every German has ready access to a doctor, cheap prescription drugs, dental care and nursing home or home health care when it is needed. All of this, and Germany spends a little more than half what the United States spends per person. Even so, their cost is one of the highest in Europe and reflects their use of the latest technology. Every facet of the health care system is on a budget, including what doctors and hospitals can charge. The "sick societies" sell all of the insurance and all of their companies are non-profit, providing more savings.

Every patient has a plastic card similar to a credit card. It is swiped through a machine when a service is performed and the information is transferred immediately to the payment center. A bill for the patient fee is sent to the person's residence and paid electronically from his or her bank account within a period of two weeks, saving billions of dollars in bookkeeping and billing over our system. Patients have a choice between taking a low-cost generic drug or a higher-priced one in the same category. The sick society pays the full cost of the generic drug and the patient pays the difference for the more expensive drug when it is chosen.

Patients have the option to enroll in a "family physician care mode." General practice physicians usually work solo, while physicians in hospitals work as teams. Patients can be referred to specialists by their regular care providers or they can go directly to the specialists. Compensation for medical personnel is negotiated annually on a regional basis between the non-profit insurance companies and medical association representatives. According to the World Health

Organization, there are 358.4 doctors per 100,000 citizens, a number considered adequate.

Medical education is provided by state universities. Unlike our system, German medical students begin their studies the first year of college. The study extends through four years of graduate school. Until recently, there were no costs to medical students or to students in any other subject for education in Germany. The Supreme Court has now ruled that states have the right to impose fees if they chose and many universities make modest charges. Now it may cost a few thousand dollars to get a complete college and medical education.

The German system is always considered to be a work in progress. Health reform is a constant topic in German federal politics. Germany is creating an agency to determine effectiveness of new drugs relative to existing ones, taking into account their relative costs. They are also working to standardize medical treatment based on proven best results.

Germany blends a private/public regulated health care delivery system with universal coverage and social solidarity in that every citizen has complete access to all services without respect to income or social status. Coverage is portable and persons are always covered. No family ever goes bankrupt over health care bills. Persons with chronic illness pay an upper limit of 1% of their income for health care.

The Health Care System of France

The World Health Organization (WHO) in 2001 chose France as the world's best health care system. WHO explained the criteria for the evaluation: coverage is universal, the health care providers are well-trained and responsive to patient needs, there is freedom for both doctors and patients, and empirical evidence shows that France is a healthy nation where the citizens live a long time.

The system is one of the most costly in Europe with a per capita cost of $3,500 in 2008 and an expenditure of 11% of the gross domestic product. That is still a bargain as compared to the United States, which spent an average of $7,300 per person the same year on health care. Every type of expenditure in the French public system is monitored and controlled, whereas here costs are what the market will bear, most of which is beyond the control of individual patients or the government. Practically all physicians in France participate in the national system called "Securité Sociale." The average American physician's salary is about three times that of the average American worker whereas the average French doctor makes about two times as much as the average Frenchman. Yet there are always more young people seeking to get into medical schools than there are openings. Medical school is offered free of charge for students, so students do not enter practice with a backlog of debt. Also, medical malpractice claims are limited and malpractice insurance is inexpensive because of the tort-adverse legal system. There are 337 doctors per 1,000 of population.

The amount doctors can charge is negotiated between the physicians' union and the public health insurance companies. 56% of doctors work in private practice while 36% of physicians are on salary working for the government in hospitals. Hospitals are owned and operated by the states. Health authorities plan the size and number of hospitals. They also decide the amount and type of medical technology that is used.

The federal health insurance program covers 99.9% of the population. Enrollment is mandatory. Doctors and hospitals can be either public or private. A doctor chooses which system to join. A physician in private practice may charge more for services and offer nicer décor in his office or a shorter time in the waiting room. Wealthier people and corporate executives usually choose a private provider. Some private hospitals, usually in the larger cities, are new, have more of the latest technology, and offer private rooms for which they set their own rates. They collect the same amount from the government as do the public hospitals, and the patient pays the additional cost out-of-pocket.

Health insurance is paid via employers. 83% of the population is insured through their employers, with special programs for the self-employed, agriculture workers, and others. Typically, the employer pays 13.55% of salary into an insurance fund and the worker adds 0.75%. In addition, the federal government adds a subsidy of 5%, making a total of 18.55%. But that is not all. The French believe the patient should have a stake in the system. The patient pays 30% of the bill for outpatient services. They pay a smaller slice of hospital costs for up to 30 days of care, but nothing beyond that limit. Patients with a chronic illness pay nothing for their care, nor do those whose income is below a set level. There is no stigma on the poor who are never considered as "means tested." 92% of the population take out supplementary private insurance to pay their 30% share, much like many of our seniors on Medicare buy a supplement to fill in the gaps. It is against the law to drop a subscriber of supplemental insurance because of a major illness. There are a wide variety of providers in the private supplemental market offering an extensive range of plans to meet individual circumstances. The patient chooses the type of plan and the amount of supplemental coverage he or she can afford and needs, all on a basic foundation of government benefits.

Typically, patients pay the full cost of treatment at the time of delivery. Their local health insurance departments reimburse them promptly for the covered expenses. All French citizens carry computerized Smart Cards containing all needed information, including their medical records. Every person in the country, including those present illegally or as visitors, has a right to health care under the French system. In the past, all EU expats coming to France were eligible to join the healthcare system immediately. However, now those who are retired, or have their healthcare costs covered by their own country, will not be allowed to join the system for five years. Until then, they can purchase private insurance and use the system.

How well do the French people like their system? The Deloitte Center for Health Solutions was commissioned to do a national survey in 2010 to answer that question. For the first time a scientific study was aimed at determining French health care attitudes, behaviors, and unmet needs. 92% of users say they are moderately or completely satisfied with their health care system. 31% rate their physical health as "excellent" or "very good", 43% as "good" and 25% as "fair" or "poor."

People want the system to do more to promote wellness, although more than a third report they make a serious effort to manage weight, eat a healthy diet, get adequate exercise, reduce stress, and be socially connected to others. 58% report a strong interest in joining a healthy living/wellness program, if it were offered at no cost. About that same percent like the idea of their insurance offering rewards for smoking cessation, weight loss, and fitness programs. Most respondents believe these programs would more than pay for themselves in reduced health care costs.

64% of recently hospitalized people say they were satisfied with the care they received. Most favor hospitals that specialize in the services they need. 94% of French citizens have a primary care physician. Overall, satisfaction is high and physician switching is rare. Enrollees are free to change doctors, but they must report the change to a state office.

A survey was conducted among those who get services from private clinics. Of these only 15% believe the quality of care is better than that provided in public clinics. 20% say they use private care because they don't want to wait for lab tests and appointments, as they sometimes do in the public clinics.

11% are likely to choose a doctor who integrates holistic or alternative treatments into their practice. The same percentage of respondents prefers a natural therapy to a prescription drug, and 10% have combined a natural treatment with a drug regimen. The French system accepts alternative therapies as legitimate and pays for them. Both the patient and the attending physician must agree that the treatment is appropriate and may offer a better path to restored health.

France still has the tradition of families caring for their ill and elderly members. 14% of French people say they provide constant care-giving for a family member. 41% of these caregivers report providing care for more than two years. 51% of these say this role reduces their ability to earn income. Slightly more than half of these caregivers are between ages 18 and 44.

Public policy issues currently being debated include expanding community services such as home care, day programs for the elderly and meals on wheels. A second is the issue of increased funding for public health surveillance and quicker response to potential disease outbreaks. Third is how government can do a better job by using complete electronic health records more effectively. It is clear that French people do not want major changes in their system. They do want constant upgrading with minor changes to make it more efficient and to improve quality.

Health Care System of the United Kingdom

The National Health Service (NHS) began operations in 1948, following the law's passage in 1946. NHS embraced the principle of collective responsibility for health care, along with a national commitment to equal access. The political consensus was forged during World War II, when all strata of society fought and often died together for the preservation of the nation. **The British people decided that access to good health care was an inherent right of every citizen.**

The United Kingdom is comprised of four countries: England, Scotland, Wales and Northern Ireland, with a total population of 60 million. 89% of the people live in urban areas. NHS is a single national system in which government owns and operates virtually all of the hospitals and pays all providers. 99+% of the people are covered by the system; those not registered are homeless people who live in private shelters. Each country has its own health ministry, with administration and control within each country under the UK umbrella. Over the years each country has evolved distinctive policies and outlooks.

Initially, physicians were wary of joining the National Health Service. They sought to preserve the right to private practice and demanded control over most medical decisions. In the end their representatives negotiated with government authorities and agreed on a plan in which they would become independent contractors. They insisted on more national control of policies vs. local control and they received the right to private practice. However, they agreed to work for a set annual fee. Similarly, all hospital medical personnel, including specialists, nurses, and technicians, are paid an annual salary.

Doctors may also have private patients who are paid beyond their regular salaries, and this can be covered by private health insurance. However, as a whole, people are satisfied with their public system and private plans are quite minimal.

Total expenditures on health care are 6.7% of GDP, lower than the Western Europe average of 8.5%. In fact, by this measure the U.K. ranks 20th among 21 industrialized countries. This low cost indicates the most efficient system or the one with the lowest quality of care. British people believe theirs is most efficient with government owning or controlling all of its parts. The government provides 85% of the total cost of all health expense, among the highest share of total health care expense in Western Europe. This leaves a low level of private spending on health care in the U.K.

Each country within the NHS system uses General Practitioners (GPs) to provide primary health care and make referrals for further service as needed. Hospitals then provide more specialized services, including care for patients with psychiatric illnesses. Pharmacies are privately owned but have contracts with the relevant health service to supply prescription drugs at a predetermined price.

Each country's public healthcare system provides free ambulance service for emergency care as needed. Dental services are provided through private practices but dentists can only charge NHS patients at a set rate that varies from one country to the next. However, about half of dentist income in England comes from their subcontracts with the NHS but not all dentists choose to do NHS work.

Health care services are available 24 hours a day. Nationwide, there are 24-hour telephone advisory services available to guide persons with sudden illnesses or accidents.

The National Institute for Health and Clinical Excellence (NICE) sets guidelines for medical practitioners as to how various conditions should be treated, and sets guidelines on what services the system will fund.

Patients may select their doctors, although they must choose one within the area where they reside. People seldom change their GP, unless they move to a new location or feel they need the guidance of a doctor who is a specialist in their illness. This system has the advantage of doctor and patient knowing each other over many years.

There are approximately 28,000 general practitioners in 9,000 practices, with an average of three doctors per practice. New practices can be set up in areas designated as "open" by the central Medical Practice Committee. Other areas are "restricted" because the supply of doctors is already sufficient in those areas. There are 300 physicians per 100,000 of population, lower than in most European countries. However, nurses and other trained medical technicians go to people's homes and provide part of the care usually reserved for doctors in other countries.

The doctor is not paid a salary but receives a gross income as an independent self-employed professional, under a "cost plus" principle. The income is negotiated for three years at the national level between the British Medical Association and the Department of Health. General Practitioners receive four types of payment:

1. Capita fees. This income for each registered patient amounts to just over half the total received. It

includes bonuses for getting superior results from treatments.

2. Allowances. This fee is paid for the cost of setting up and managing the practice.

3. Health Promotion payments. Additional amounts are paid to the doctor for services such as promoting wellness programs, administering chronic disease treatments, or providing childhood immunizations.

4. Items of Source Payment. A relatively small number of negotiated items, such as providing birth control services, make up this category.

Hospital doctors negotiate separately for their compensation packages via their medical association. Specialists who have had additional years of training receive somewhat higher incomes. They can have some private patients and earn up to 10% beyond their regular compensation packages. Hospital doctors can also get merit awards for outstanding service.

Nurses are trained for one of three types of setting. "Practice nurses" are employed by GPs and work within practices. They manage chronic diseases, administer vaccines and other routine procedures and make home visits to the elderly. There are 10,000 nurses of this type. Another type is the "community nurse." These nurses are employed by community hospitals. They often do outreach, going to the homes of patients who find it hard to travel to the hospital or doctor's office. This category includes midwives and various types of therapists. Another 10,000 fall into this category. Finally, there are official "health visitors" who take over from midwives. They specialize in serving families with babies and young children. The midwife who has served the woman during her pregnancy continues to go to the home and work with mother and baby for 28 days and then the health visitor takes over with a focus on wellness, good nutrition and good principles of child rearing. About 12,000 of these nurses are on active duty.

There are about 10,000 pharmacies in the United Kingdom that dispense drugs prescribed by physicians. The price of each drug is set by negotiations between the government and the drug manufacturer. However, the number of drugs being prescribed continues to grow and this is causing policy concern. The government is expanding the role of pharmacists, authorizing them to counsel clients, check to make sure clients are not taking drugs that adversely interact, and offer policy recommendations on drug-related issues.

Medical education and nursing education are provided at public expense. The medical student usually does a five year undergraduate degree with a major in medical studies in one of 19 medical schools, each part of a university. The next year is spent in a hospital as an intern, supervised by the college medical program. If the student passes and is going into General Practice, he or she continues to study in a hospital for another five years, while gaining practical experience. Those going into specialties, including surgery, continue to study under supervision for an additional two years. Every physician is required to participate in a lifelong learning program. Medical students are paid by the Higher Education Funding Council while they are in training.

Hospitals get 69% of their income from block grants, depending on the number of people in their district. 25% is based on the actual volume of patients, while 5% relates to the cost per patient served. Only rarely is payment based on an individual fee for service.

Each country is divided into districts, with a General Hospital in each district. This is the backbone of the hospital system. It was introduced in the 1960s to provide comprehensives services for between 150,000 and 200,000 residents at each hospital. The model remains intact. Outpatient clinics and outreach into the community are based in the hospital.

Two other types of hospital complete the system. Regional hospitals are larger and offer more specializations. Community hospitals have up to 200 beds, but more typically 50 beds, and provide routine operations. Most also provide day care services for the elderly. These hospitals are often favored by users and the government, as they are closer to home and are less expensive to operate when patients do not require more intensive services.

In addition to the public system, a small number of private hospitals exist. They also receive public funds based on the national formula, but they offer more upscale settings and some additional services for which patients pay extra. Public hospitals also offer some special "amenity" beds. Clients pay extra for private rooms with upscale services. Only 3% of GPs choose full-time private practice.

In 1991 the General Hospitals became National Trusts with the expectation that they would generate income above their expenditures. A 6% return on investment was posited. Now the clinics within hospitals are often contracted to private groups who pay rent for the space. The hospital Administrator coordinates and directs all of the clinics. The Trusts are independent from the National Health System. They are non-profit, and the income they generate is used to pay for new technology, renovation of buildings, and similar expenses.

Each country must decide how to care for its elderly and chronically ill citizens who need special assistance. Great Britain uses five million "independent contractors," some of whom work part-time. These caregivers work in private homes, local government-operated assisted living or nursing homes and in privately operated assisted living facilities. Money is allotted to local health departments that hire and train care givers and supervise the services they provide.

Persons with adequate wealth are no longer eligible for senior public assistance. An issue being debated is whether the elderly should have to sell their family home and use the money before becoming eligible for public assistance.

Constant attention is paid to improving the health care system, formalized through a national "Institute for Innovation and Improvement" that researches new technologies and techniques. After experimental programs are tried and proved successful, the Institute helps set up training programs that spread the knowledge widely among all health care providers. Hospital and GP doctors are surveyed regularly on the procedures they use, and patients are surveyed on their health care experiences.

Medical groups are compared with their peers in other locations to assess what treatments and procedures produce the best outcomes. Since 2005, efficiency of organization has been a factor in determining payment levels for GPs.

Generally, the people of the United Kingdom are proud of their health care system. When the Conservative government comes into power, it tinkers around the edges and introduces minor private sector changes. The nation remains united in the conviction that every citizen must be fully covered with the best medical care available, and that it is the responsibility of society as a whole to pay for this fundamental right. **By centralizing administration, eliminating duplication and controlling cost at every level, the United Kingdom has achieved quality care at lower cost than 18 other countries of Europe and at less than half of the per person cost in the United States.**

The Health Care System of Japan

Universal health care is enshrined in the Japanese constitution. The system traces its beginning to a textile company that introduced health insurance to its employees in 1905. A broad health insurance law for employees was passed in 1922 inspired by the German model. In 1927 the law was extended to cover individuals not receiving health insurance from an employer. Since 1961 virtually every person has been guaranteed access to all health services. The Japanese system is well tested and widely appreciated by the great majority of people. Those who cannot afford the premiums are subsidized by public funds.

In 2008 Japan's health care cost $2,581 per person while ours had a price tag of $7,290. The Japanese government paid out 8.1% of its gross domestic product for health care, compared with our 16%. But, some respond, we provide better medicine, better hospitals and more advanced medical care. Not true. Japanese citizens live longer on average than we do. The number of infants lost at childbirth is 2.6 per thousand while we lose 6.7 per thousand. By almost any measure the Japanese excel us in health care outcomes, although we have an almost equal percentage of doctors; they have 610 per thousand population and we have 611. One cultural factor that affects cost involves Japan's significantly lower need for emergency room services. While Japan has half the population of our country, they suffer only seven percent of the murders, one percent of the rapes, 0.3 percent of armed robberies, and a tiny fraction of the stabbings and gunshot wounds, so they have relatively little need for trauma facilities. This represents a significant cost saving.

Japan has a complex system of 2,000 private insurance companies and 3,000 units of government that all have a role in the health care system. However, the system can be reduced to two broad categories: (1) 65% of the population gets coverage from their employers, including their dependents, and (2) self-employed persons and their dependents, the unemployed, and the elderly are covered through some form of managed government program, administered through a network of 300 local offices.

All health insurance companies in Japan are non-profit. They all cover the same services and offer drugs for the same price. The Japanese Health Ministry has a 20-person Council representing a cross-section of society that controls prices and negotiates rates with the health care industry and the drug companies every two years. These uniform prices form an implicit global budget the country relies on to control their health care expenditures.

Doctors and hospitals function in the private sector of the economy. Patients choose their doctors and have access to all doctors and hospitals. They have the option to go directly to a hospital without a referral from a general practitioner. Japanese physicians practice as individuals or in small-scale clinics. They often have their offices in their own residences. Small outpatient clinics have traditionally provided most outpatient care. Local inpatient clinics have up to 19 beds and function as small hospitals. They compete actively with larger hospitals for patients.

Until the late 1980s there were few barriers placed on entry to the hospital market. 81% of hospitals are privately owned. They have few restrictions on capital investment. Some 90% of hospitals are classified as "general hospitals." The others specialize in mental health, cancer or tuberculosis. All hospitals are operated as "non-profit" facilities. The average private hospital has 163 beds. The 19% operated by a government entity average 283 beds and account for a third of the total. All hospital medical personnel are salaried.

Hospitals have traditionally functioned also as recuperative and long-term care facilities as needed. This is due largely to the small size of Japanese houses and the fact that bedrooms serve as common rooms during the day. The average number of days in the hospital is longer in Japan than in any other country in the world. 75% of institutionalized elderly are in hospitals and clinics. 45% of the elderly who go to the hospital stay for more than six months. Nursing homes and assisted living facilities are just now gaining traction and some persons needing extra care are moving from hospitals to these facilities.

A Medicare equivalent kicks in for the elderly at age 70, or at age 65 if persons are incapacitated, bedridden or not able to care for themselves. The federal government pays half the cost from general funds and the remainder is paid by a dedicated tax on all employed persons.

What does the citizen pay and how much is covered in a typical health insurance plan? The patient pays up to 30% of the cost for routine visits to the doctor and for prescription drugs. When the cost is considered catastrophic or the person cannot afford to pay, government provides service without cost to the patient. Government or the employer pays 81% of the total cost of all health care. In the employment sector, employers pay some 96% of insurance premium costs and employees add the final 4%.

Coverage is complete except for routine physicals, some types of dental work and over-the-counter drugs. The coverage includes hospital in-patient and out-patient care, home care, cost of childbirth plus cash benefits, dental, prescriptions, long-term care in a facility or home care when it is more beneficial, and medical devices that enhance living. Maternity leave for 100 days is compensated at 50% of the mother's salary. The approach used in Japan provides one of the most efficient systems in the world at low cost and high quality.

The Health Care System of Sweden

Matt Yglesias quotes an official Swedish government source on the philosophy behind Sweden's health care system: **"Swedish health and medical care is based on the principles that care should be provided on equal terms and according to need; that it should be under democratic control and financed on the basis of solidarity."** [35]

Everyone in Sweden has equal access to health care services.   The Swedish health care system is largely taxpayer funded and decentralized. The role of the central government is to establish guidelines for care and to set the political agenda for medical services. Beyond overarching laws, the central government coordinates agreements with the Swedish Association of Local Authorities and Regions, which represents the county councils and municipalities.

Responsibility for providing health care is decentralized to the county councils and to municipal governments in the cities. County councils and cities elect candidates from their jurisdictions who serve four year terms. They are elected when national general elections are held. No hierarchical structure exists among counties, municipalities or regions. Each has certain responsibilities that do not overlap with other jurisdictions.

Sweden's municipalities are responsible for the care of elderly people in their homes or in special accommodations. They also care for people with physical disabilities and psychological disorders. They provide support services for patients as they are released from hospitals.   Finally, they provide health care services for children in schools.

Most of the responsibility for care falls on the 18 County Councils who provide for the people residing in their jurisdiction.   People receive primary health care in just over 1,000 "health centers," where general practitioners work in clusters with nurses, therapists, midwives, home health aides, and other providers. Patients are free to choose their GP. Each center must provide emergency health service until 9 p.m.   There are separate clinics for children and expecting mothers, as well as different youth clinics, that offer advice to that age group on a range of issues, including family planning.

There are 70 county hospitals and eight regional hospitals in Sweden.   County hospitals are under the control of county governments. The eight larger regional hospitals treat more specialized illnesses. They, too, are owned by the counties where they are located. They are focal points for research and for the training of medical personnel.   Obviously, every county does not have a regional hospital, so counties that lack a regional hospital pay to use the closest one in a county that does.

At an earlier time more patient care was done in the hospital setting. As it became evident that it costs less to treat patients in health centers, much of the medical work formerly done in hospitals was transferred there. Many large hospitals still offer general patient care, however, and a hospital is never far from where a patient lives.

71% of the cost of health care provided by a county is financed by county taxes. The patient also pays a small amount at the time of treatment, and the remainder is covered from national taxes. Patient payments are charged to give patients a stake in the cost and encourage the person to go to a GP rather than a hospital for treatment. Out-of-pocket costs per person are capped at $125 annually.

In 2005 the total health care spending for everything, including eye glasses, was 9.1 percent of GDP, compared to the 16+% for the United States, a figure that has remained fairly stable since the mid 1980s. These costs are on par with those of most other European countries. Life expectancy has been rising steadily. In 2008 it was age 79 for men and 83 for women.

The primary criticism of the system has been that there is often a significant wait for elective surgery, such as cataract or hip-replacement surgery. Sweden introduced a health care guarantee in 2005. It declared that no patient should have to wait more than 90 days. If the time limit expires in a given county, patients are offered care in another. The cost, including travel and housing for accompanying family, is paid by the County Council where the patient resides. To improve the situation still more, the Swedish Association of Local Authorities and Regions decided to allocate an extra $140 million U.S. equivalent each year between 2010 and 2012 to alleviate shortages and then evaluate to determine a more permanent solution.

Sweden has introduced an element of private care into the system. County councils may buy services from private health care providers. 10% of health care financed by county councils is now carried out by these private providers.   An agreement guarantees that patients are covered by the same regulations and fees as those paid in the public system.

Costs are controlled in every aspect of the system. Standard salaries are paid to doctors, nurses, medical specialists, therapists and all other providers. The national government negotiates rates for cost of drugs and lower cost generic drugs are used when appropriate.   All hospitals are government owned and operated on a non-profit basis.

The Health Care System of Canada

Canada has universal coverage for its citizens. Their plan is funded and administered through government entities in a shared federal/provincial system. The plan does not provide for all costs, but the government pays for the entire cost of care that is provided through the plan. Persons may buy private insurance policies to fill in the gaps, much as our seniors can get supplemental insurance with their Medicare policies.

Patients choose their doctors, who are private providers.   Hospitals are both publicly and privately owned, but government pays all hospital costs for patients. Government negotiates for the price of drugs, driving down prices to the point where drug companies receive a moderate but fair compensation.

Coverage for patients includes all medically necessary hospital and physician services, but not dental care, out-patient prescription drugs or rehab services. Private supplemental insurance can be purchased to cover these costs. Patients do not have to bother with co-payments or deductibles.

The federal government sets national standards, determines prices that will be paid, and gives the financial support. Each of the provincial and territorial governments is responsible for administering the single-payer system for universal medical and hospital services in the region. Private insurance is prohibited by law from covering the same benefits as the public plan.

Federal and provincial taxes cover 70% of the total cost of insurance and individuals pay the remainder. Most of these government insurance funds are collected through income taxes, but sales taxes and payroll taxes also contribute.

The Canadian system, known as Medicare, covers the entire population and performs well as a single-payer system. Strong federal regulation of cost creates a system that provides universal coverage at lower costs than in the United States. The system has often been slow to schedule elective surgeries for conditions that are not considered life-threatening. It is this aspect of the Canadian system that is most heavily criticized by opponents in the United States.

A Final Summary

Each of these health care systems operates more efficiently and effectively than ours, with lower costs and better outcomes. Each country is proud of what it has achieved and would not consider returning to an uncontrolled system in which private providers skim off large profits and charge whatever the market will bear.

Most consider it a crime against humanity to force the poor to go without medical treatment, drive vulnerable people into bankruptcy, or gouge the system for private gain at public expense. There is no place for the health care lobbying empire that operates in Washington, D.C. A final mark of these health care systems is they are not too proud to learn from each other.

All other advanced countries pay the cost of medical education for every type of provider and then pay salaries rather than fees for services. Each country has a waiting list of young people wanting to spend their lives helping others in the field of medicine. Every country recognizes that its system is never complete or perfect. Rather, it must be constantly reviewed, studied and updated for better medicine, better delivery and better cost management.

Chapter 6

MORAL ISSUES

"The moral arc of the universe leans toward justice."
—Martin Luther King, Jr.

A man died, according to the story, and awoke in hell. There he saw men and women gathered around tables filled with delicious food and drink; yet the people were starving and thirsty. They could not feed themselves, because metal rods kept their arms straight and prevented them from lifting food and drink to their mouths. Later, that same man was transported to heaven. There he witnessed the same scene. Men and women were gathered around tables overflowing with good food and drink. The same metal rods were strapped to their arms, yet in heaven all of the people were well fed and happy. What was the difference between hell and heaven? In hell, people were thinking only of themselves. Since they couldn't bend their arms, they couldn't get food or drink. They were miserable, on the verge of starvation. In heaven, the people were feeding each other. By being concerned for the other and by working together, all were well fed.

As Americans, we all have values that form our core beliefs. We apply these values to our assessment of the Affordable Care Act. We do so explicitly by consciously thinking about the issues or implicitly by our unconscious assumptions.

Our American psyche has two deep-seated values that appear to be in conflict. They are contained in our Pledge of Allegiance: "...with liberty and justice for all."

"Liberty" implies the freedom to go our own way, to be independent and self-reliant. The free enterprise economic system that we enjoy is a direct expression of our liberty. We have an inherent right, we believe, to choose our own jobs, decide how hard we want to work, start our own businesses, invent creative ways to make money, invest as we see fit, and prosper accordingly.

"Justice for all" is a recognition that we live in community, and that our individual freedom does not give us license to pursue our interests to the detriment of others. In that awareness, our constitution was framed to provide for "the general welfare." Our vision of fairness does not demand that every person have equal pay with every other person. It does require a social and economic system in which people's financial rewards are reasonably proportional to their contributions to an economic endeavor. Those with the greatest social and economic leverage should not be able to game the system and siphon off most of the rewards, leaving other stakeholders without enough money to live decently and without health care security. We strive for every child to have an equal opportunity to develop his or her potential, regardless of parents' socioeconomic status. Within our national social contract we believe that every person has rights. The dignity and needs of every person are to be respected. There should be justice for all.

These two values of liberty and justice have existed side by side since our nation was founded. Rather than affirm that one is right and the other is wrong, many of us insist that both are vitally important, even though they always exist together in dynamic tension. It is not "either, or" but rather "both, and." A "good society" must uphold both. Our plight is always to wrestle with the relative importance of these two fundamental values, while affirming both. **Many of us believe the modern political right values unfettered "liberty" at the expense of justice.**

There are always boundaries to be placed on liberty. Liberty is never an excuse to "do as you please." Liberty always rests within a matrix of responsibility. Do as you please within the context of "the common good." In the realm of the free enterprise business system, liberty does not mean "get what you can" without regard to the social, environmental, and other consequences of your actions. Too many free market corporate and Wall Street types—armed with their unlimited access to money for politicians and willfully oblivious to the systemic effects of their actions —proclaim that "greed is good," and what is good for the ultra-wealthy is good for the country. They make their appeal by associating their actions and attendant propaganda with the ideal of "freedom." Politicians call for freedom from regulation in the critical health care field as part of their allegiance to "liberty" without considering the damage predatory practices can cause to the common good.

Our Current Health Care Dilemma

Our health care costs are soaring. Each year millions more Americans lose health insurance. Millions more keep insurance but do so at the expense of other basic living needs. Business is losing its competitive edge because of the high cost of health insurance. Our per capita cost of health care is almost double that of any other country in the world. How can we respond morally to this dilemma?

We begin with the recognition, again, that some areas of our common life are best served by private entrepreneurship, by the free market with appropriate regulation where needed. In other areas we are served best by a more communal approach. Put another way, private enterprise best serves our interests in most areas, but in others, government is required to provide for and protect the general welfare. We can employ a judicious mixture of private and public in health care, but the public interest must trump private profit and poor health care outcomes. Our health care is an area too important to leave to random market forces and the manipulations of powerful corporate interests.

We reject the notion that each person is an island, responsible only for self. Government is not best that governs least in the vital area of health care. We are all vulnerable to accident and sickness, and it is our common destiny to die. Do we identify with our common humanity, our common experiences of good health, sickness and death? **The Affordable Care Act reflects a vision that every American has a right to good medical care. This law commits us to work together to develop and refine a health care system that benefits everyone.**

When we stop to consider carefully, we realize that all insurance is communal. Insurance spreads risk. Even though some people in any insurance pool always end up paying more than they get in claims, everyone benefits by limiting their risk. In the case of health insurance, we eliminate the chance that health care costs could bankrupt all but the richest among us. In a health insurance policy most of us pay more into a plan than we receive back. Indeed, we are the lucky ones if we don't need to use the health care system much. Some of us get back more than we pay in. That is the way the social contract works: We pay to help ourselves and other people, and others pay to help us in our hour of need. All benefit by limiting risk.

The Committed Opposition

The "committed opposition" to the Affordable Care Act wants to keep health care in the private sector to the extent possible. Two perspectives dominate the landscape. First, there is the minority that prefers to exclude government from any involvement in health care. For them, "that government is best that governs least." Their vision is to turn loose the free enterprise system so that people can have the dignity to sink or swim, depending on their own resourcefulness. They do see a role for the religious community and other private organizations to assist the poor. When Congressman Ron Paul was asked in a Republican debate whether he would just let people die if they had no money to pay the hospital bill, many in the audience cheered. But Mr. Paul said he didn't expect that would happen. Church groups would step in and pay the bill! With the cost of an average hospital stay at well beyond $20,000, one has trouble envisioning the average parish paying for more than one or two hospitalizations per year.

While it is true that some inner-city churches, synagogues, and mosques now have health clinics and other outreach programs that serve the poor in their areas—and this is a valuable contribution—in our modern, complex society, government is the only entity large enough and comprehensive enough to effectively address our needs. Private charities and religious organizations help thousands, while only government can serve the needs of millions. All charitable efforts combined are not large enough to make a significant dent in the total need. A recent study by two sociologists, Mark Chaves of Duke University and Bob Wineburg at the University of North Carolina, Greensboro, led them to conclude, "National and local studies make clear that congregations occupy an important but limited place in community social service systems."[36]

Another prominent position held by "pre-tea party" Republicans is to leave each person to fend for himself or herself in getting medical insurance, but when a medical emergency arises, government should require hospitals to treat the sick even if they can't pay. These Republicans and a minority of Democrats believe society has an obligation to provide a minimum safety net, if only to keep people from dying in the streets. This, for them, is the limit of public responsibility; they deny universal coverage as a social obligation. In fact, the most generous Republican health plan offered thus far covered only four million additional persons, while the Affordable Care Act passed by Democrats covered an additional thirty-two million Americans.

David Brooks, in his new book *The Social Animal: the Hidden Sources of Love, Character and Achievement* (The New York Times, 2011), drives home the point that we are not basically individuals first who then develop social relationships, but rather we are social beings who later become individuals. We learn from others—our language, our values and all the rest that we know—as we gradually grow into unique persons. We are humble and grateful when we acknowledge we would hardly be human were it not for the care and concern freely given to us when we could not provide for ourselves. We are most fully human when we live with compassion and concern and give back to the entire community.

Various estimates are made as to the number of persons who die each year from lack of proper medical care, mostly for financial reasons. A 2009 Harvard Study published in the *American Journal of Public Health* found 49,000 deaths annually "associated with lack of insurance."[37]

Some of us choose to see health care as a basic human right. We reject the morality of a public policy of "pay or die" that makes life dependent upon being relatively wealthy, having a good job with insurance benefits, or being a member of the armed forces.

John Boehner (R. Ohio), Speaker of the House of Representatives, gave the 2011 commencement address to the graduating class at Catholic University of America.[38] According to E. J. Dionne, Jr., "He offered a sweet-natured, non-political talk about the power of humility, patience and faith, complete with references to the Blessed Mother, the Hail Mary prayer, and the speaker's intrepid Catholic high school football coach."

A group of Catholic academics, including many leading faculty members at Catholic University, responded with a letter to Congressman Boehner. "We congratulate you on the occasion of your commencement address at The Catholic University of America. It is good for Catholic universities to host and engage the thoughts of powerful public figures, even Catholics such as yourself who fail to recognize (whether out of lack of awareness or dissent) important aspects of Catholic teachings." The remainder of the letter was respectful but tough. "From the apostles to the present," the professors wrote, "the Magisterium of the Church has insisted that those in power are morally obligated to preference the needs of the poor." They added, "Your record in support of legislation to address the desperate needs of the poor is among the worst in Congress." The letter specifically condemned the Ryan-passed budget, arguing that it guts long-established protections for the most vulnerable members of society.

In November of 2010, Pope Joseph Ratzinger, now known as Benedict XVI, addressed the 25th annual conference of the Pontifical Council of Health Care Ministry. He said, "Health care is one of the inalienable rights of man. Justice in health care should be a priority of governments."

Again, an important official pastoral letter of the Roman Catholic Church on economic justice had this to say: "As followers of Christ, we are challenged to make a fundamental 'option for the poor'—to speak for the voiceless, to defend the defenseless, to assess life styles, policies and social institutions in terms of their impact on the poor. This 'option for the poor' does not mean pitting one group against another, but rather, strengthening the whole community by assisting those who are the most vulnerable. As Christians, we are called to respond to the needs of all our brothers and sisters, but those with the greatest needs require the greatest response."[39]

This I Believe

My basic assumptions are founded on the life and teachings of Jesus. In Matthew 28, among other places in the Christian Bible, Jesus calls us to care for the sick, the distressed, the poor and the outcast. He then said, "In as much as you did it for one of the least of these, you did it for me." Sobering words! My Episcopal Church Book of Common Prayer, in our baptismal vows, leads us to commit to "serving God in every person" and "respecting the dignity of every person." Ever since Thomas Cramer wrote the first Anglican Prayer Book in the early 17th Century, virtually every congregation of Anglicans in the world has prayed weekly for the poor.

Christians pray for the poor because they are God's children, given irreducible dignity by the endless love of God. Whatever else we say about citizens without health insurance, Christians are compelled to say these are God's children. They have a special place in the heart of God precisely because they are poor and without resources such as health care. Biblical faith reveals a "strategic concentration" of love for the underprivileged. God sees their affliction. God knows their suffering. God does not will that one of these should perish. So the Christian Bible proclaims.

Jesus summarized the essential teaching behind all of the Hebrew laws and the basic message of prophets across hundreds of years: "You shall love the Lord your God with all of your heart, with all of your soul, with all of your strength, and with all of your mind. And the second command is like the first, you shall love your neighbor as yourself" (Luke 10:25-37). The question that followed is the one asked in every age since Jesus, "Who is my neighbor?"

Jesus told the story of the "Good Samaritan" as his answer. A despised stranger travelling from another country sees a wounded man at the roadside, carries him to an inn where he can get treatment, and pays the cost of that care. Those we do not know personally are still neighbors, and we are accountable for their well-being. They may be travelers or immigrants in our country, injured or abandoned people, perhaps of a different religion. They are all neighbors when they are in need.

It is in this spirit that I support the Affordable Care Act and want to work tirelessly for its preservation and improvement. I am reminded of the question asked of us in John's epistle, "How does God's love abide in us who have this world's goods when we see brothers and sisters in need, and yet refuse to help?"[40]

Some of my fellow Christians feel that individual salvation through the death and resurrection of Jesus is more important than any "social gospel." My response is, "In your effort to promote a plan of salvation, please don't at the same time fail to focus on the humanity of Jesus and his years of teaching, healing and giving preferential treatment to the poor and others without power. Please do not diminish his supreme teaching to "love your neighbor as yourself."

Another aspect of Christian responsibility from my perspective is truth-telling. It involves debunking the powerful, complex myth that has grown up around national health insurance. Many Americans claim and repeat endlessly that: (1) the Affordable Care Act would be too expensive—it might even bankrupt the country; (2) it would take away people's choice of doctors; (3) it would necessarily cause long waits for care; (4) it would inappropriately ration health care; or (5) it just wouldn't work because government can't do anything right.

None of this need be true. None of this characterizes the health care systems of other countries. All industrial democracies except ours provide universal coverage, better health outcomes, and far lower costs than we do. Now Medicare provides for most of the health needs of all Americans over age 65 at a 3% overhead. It is not beyond human intelligence or the "can do" American spirit to design a health care system that is morally responsible.

I believe that as a Christian I cannot divorce myself from this critical aspect of public policy. At the same time, I cannot impose my understanding of Christian values on our pluralistic society. Rather, as a Christian citizen I work with those who share my values to influence the political debate. Most other religions and secular approaches to morality share concern for the poor and an appreciation for the common good.

Other Moral Perspectives

The Hebrew scripture calls for social justice that serves the interests of the poor, a society where people care for each other. When the poor suffer because of injustice or insensitivity, "I will surely hear their cry. My anger will burn...."(Exodus 22:22). Whatever my theological differences with my Jewish friends, I stand ready to join hands with them in designing a system that meets the health care needs of every person. We join hands and hearts at a profound level, where we share our belief in a God who demands justice and is equally concerned for everyone.

Islam repeatedly turns to the Holy Qur'an to explain what it means to be religious. Allah makes it clear that piety has two dimensions. The first consists of worship and prayer. The other is social in nature and comprises our obligation to society, particularly to the disadvantaged. Indeed, every Muslim is taught that the community has a stake in whatever the Muslim owns. A good Muslim purifies himself or herself from greed and excessive materialism and helps build a strong society.

And, yes, there are millions of "secular humanists" who are not primarily inspired by religious faith. Many non-religious people value human dignity and have well-developed moral sensibilities. We unite in our efforts to see that all of our citizens have quality health care at a price we as a society can afford. We are equally committed to working for the common good.

Secular humanists can look to Plato, one of the great moral philosophers of the ages, for moral moorings. Plato said we all act out of self-love or "eros" love. But, he said, there are two kinds of eros: "vulgar" eros and "heavenly" eros. Vulgar self-love treats each person as an object to be manipulated to satisfy one's desires regardless of the effects on the other. A person operating with vulgar eros uses power to take advantage of the one who is weaker, even if it degrades that person. In economic terms, a system with underlying values based on vulgar eros encourages people to build their own personal and business wealth any way they can, without taking into account the broader consequences of their actions. Their actions often limit or reduce the wealth of those with fewer resources. That wealth is transferred to the pockets of the powerful few. This short-sighted, limited vulgar love takes advantage of others' limited ability to protect their interests. Vulgar eros seeks favored status in health care, preferring to exclude the poor with the hope that the arrangement will make their own insurance less expensive. "Greed is good" is the creed of those who live by vulgar eros.

Then, there is heavenly eros. It considers the long-term good and the broader good for everyone involved, rather than just immediate self-satisfaction. It asks, "What is the common good?" It believes that respect for the other and the long term common good are ultimately in one's own best self-interest, from this broader perspective. It is self-love for mature humans. The good society, said Plato, is one built on heavenly eros. Martin Luther King Jr. spoke with the conviction that heavenly eros is the only enduring morality when he observed, "The moral arc of the universe leans toward justice."

Whether our sense of morality is rooted in our religion or in our secular humanism, we as individuals are most fully human when we live with compassion and concern for the entire community. We as a society form an honorable nation when we translate our care for each

other into a rational system of health care for every citizen. The story at the beginning of the chapter had it right. We create hell when we think of ourselves alone; we create heaven when we mutually care for each other.

Chapter 7

REPUBLICAN RESPONSE

The basic premise of Obamacare is flawed. Any effort to repair this law is like pouring a few glasses of water into a polluted river.

--Jim DeMint, U.S. Senator, S.C. February 2011 Fox News

What has been the Republican response to passage of the Affordable Care Act of 2010? The quick answer is that they have done everything possible to reverse and defeat the Act. They prefer to repeal it entirely, but until that is possible, they seek to undermine it in every possible way. They bleed money out of the law by not passing necessary appropriations. Republicans at the state level refuse to implement provisions, including the requirement to set up insurance exchanges. They petition the Courts to have the Act declared unconstitutional. In addition, they continue an endless barrage of words to discredit the law by claiming it will bankrupt the treasury or turn over the health of our parents to faceless bureaucrats. In short, Republicans and their friends in the media misstate facts, distort content and mislead the public. Their intent is to confuse people so they don't know what is in the legislation or how it can help solve our health care dilemmas.

Republican Alternatives to Medicare and Medicaid

Congressman Paul Ryan (R. Wisc.), Chairman of the Finance Committee, presented the House Budget Committee's 2012 budget that reflected the first step, he said, in returning the nation to fiscal sanity. He presented two Republican fiscal goals: to cut $4.4 trillion in spending over the next decade and to lower taxes on the very wealthy and large corporations.

The part of Mr. Ryan's vision most relevant here is the way he would end Medicare as we know it and cut Medicaid.

Traditional Medicare would end in 2022. New retirees would then lose their previously guaranteed benefits, paid in part from payroll taxes they had invested in the program during their working lives. The nation would eliminate our existing public plan and substitute private insurance. An annual voucher from the government would cover part of the cost of premiums, with seniors left to pay the difference, on average an additional $7,000 the first year. The seniors' payments would increase annually, as costs increase, while the government subsidy would remain constant. In other words, the savings to balance the federal budget would come by shifting the cost of health care from government to individual seniors.

It gets worse. The Congressional Budget Office estimates that by 2030, as costs escalate, seniors would pay 70% of health care costs from their own pockets, driving millions of lower income persons out of the system.

Further, many specialists doubt that insurance companies would voluntarily offer policies to the old and infirm with multiple illnesses. Millions of seniors with varying degrees of education and cognitive function would have to sort through an array of confusing private policies and choose the right one for their situation. Paul Ryan put it like this to make it more appealing, "Just like the way your Congressman does." Seniors as a group would be forced to pay $39 trillion more for insurance coverage over 75 years than they would under existing law. Who benefits? Health insurance companies win. They add up to 50 million additional senior customers whose rates they control under "free market" economics, and whose "high risk" policies they can cancel. Again, **private insurers under the new law will reduce their overhead and profit from an average of 25 cents down to 20 cents per dollar, while Medicare spends 3 cents per dollar**. The massively higher cost of private insurance relative to Medicare would be borne by individual seniors, who would have no collective bargaining power with the insurance corporate giants and therefore no ability to deal with the systemic problems in our health care system that are being addressed by Medicare and by the ACA.

Amazingly, the Republicans quietly included in their 2012 budget plan and longer-term projections the ACA's $500 billion of savings over its first ten years as part of their plan to save four trillion dollars. This is the height of hypocrisy, as Republicans cynically misinformed their base and incited fear in the elderly by portraying these same Medicare cost savings built into the ACA through reforms and greater efficiencies as "rationing," "death panels" and "pulling the plug on grandma." Presidential candidates on the Republican side accuse "Obamacare" of robbing the elderly of $500 billion dollars in order to support the President's health care fantasy. Nonetheless, they maintain all of this "rationing" and those "death panels"—the same $500 billion, a significant part of their proposed savings—in their own plan to lower the deficit by four trillion dollars.

Democrats respond that Medicare was created in part because insurance companies often would not insure older people at greater risk of illness and need for constant care. The vast array of cost-control measures in their plan, say the Democrats, is absent from the Republican vision after the first ten years. In fact, all three goals set forth in the Affordable Care Act are missing with Ryan's Medicare proposal: it will not provide universal coverage—even for the elderly—as is now the case; quality of medical care will decline rather than advance; and costs will continue to escalate.

Republicans have never put forward an alternative plan that even begins to deal seriously with the three goals of the Affordable Care Act. Those of us who care far more about the nation's health than we do about warfare between the political parties wish fervently that they had a serious alternative. Concerned citizens speak out, not to trash Republicans, but to seriously confront the enormous challenge facing our nation so that we can find a rational solution. Rather than ask, "How can we cut Medicare to reduce the deficit?" the Affordable Care Act asks, "How can we strengthen the quality of care while also reducing costs to keep it affordable?" **Breaking the contract for universal coverage with America's seniors—a difficult-to-insure age group—is unacceptable.**

The other big saving in Paul Ryan's "Path to Prosperity" comes through cuts in Medicaid. He would cut more than $700 billion in ten years from this program that serves as a safety net for the poor and disabled. His plan is to replace Medicaid with block grants to the states, but in smaller amounts than the government spends now on Medicaid, while ending the financing partnership between the states and the federal government. States would have great latitude in spending the money and much of it could go for programs other than Medicaid. Since the amount received would be much less than they get now, and since they would not be required to match the federal contribution, it would be left to States to decide who got cut from the rolls or how much reduction everyone in the program would get. States that have never provided adequately for their destitute would do far less under this arrangement. Rather than offering hope for adequate health care for every person, this plan cuts even the existing safety net from under the poor and the elderly.

Mr. Ryan calls his new plan a way "to strengthen the social safety net, not turn it into a hammock." He shares the belief of many in his party when he continues, "We don't want this to be a food stamp nation; we want it be a paycheck nation." The obvious inference is that society will benefit by cutting the safety net from under people. This will motivate them to get good jobs so they can buy their own insurance. Apparently, the same is true for the frail elderly who have already spent whatever life savings they had on expensive drugs, therapies and hospital bills. According to this Republican narrative, people on Medicaid are linked to welfare queens driving Cadillacs. They are working the system so that many now live in food stamp mansions and fly to Hawaii for vacations, using food stamp money. Here is the latest image: we are asked to visualize the disabled, the poor and the frail elderly lying in luxury on hammocks rather than simply being protected by safety nets!

The plan was presented to the American public with the proclamation that it is the only way to save the country from bankruptcy. Republicans actually support the poor and elderly, they say, because without these cuts a bankrupt country would not be in a position to provide any support at all!

Rep. Jeff Hensarling, (R. Texas) Chairman of the GOP Conference, said on April 15, 2011 that "Medicare, Medicaid and Social Security will bankrupt the nation." He called these programs "Ponzi schemes." He admitted, "They have been of great comfort to my parents and grandparents but they're morphing into cruel Ponzi schemes for my 9 year old daughter and 7 year olds."

Democrats responded that nobody is being misled, as in a Ponzi scheme. The Social Security Trust Fund has enough money to cover the next 35 years, with its surpluses on loan to the U. S. Treasury. Nobody doubts that it would be prudent to make adjustments sooner. Further, the Affordable Care Act has extended the life of Medicare by 10 years, while building in additional cost savings that, if done well, will result in even greater savings. Medicaid has proved to be the most efficient way to provide full health care coverage for the poor and is being expanded to cover the next tier of relatively poor people. These are rational, proven ways to serve the needs of our people.

Mitch McConnell (R. Ky.), Minority Leader of the Senate, said on Fox News Sunday, May 22, 2011, "The nation faces a choice over Medicare. We can either cut back to a voucher system and save the program for seniors, or we can go the Obama way and ration care. We need to have an adult conversation about this choice. I think most Americans would rather not let a commission of bureaucrats have the power to ration care so that our seniors are left empty-handed in old age."

Republicans like to scare seniors by claiming the ACA will ration care and ruin the health of seniors. The commission to which they refer is the Independent Payment Advisory Board with its 15 distinguished members. Beginning in 2013, their task, once again, is to look for savings in the system, most of which are discussed in the chapter on cost control. Should spending grow faster than one percent more than the rate of growth of the gross domestic product, the Commission has the authority to recommend added savings. They will search for inefficiencies, fraud and abuse, and price gouging by providers. They will study the potential for additional wellness programs. Their cost-control suggestions will be sent to Congress. Should Congress fail to override their proposed cuts with its own solutions, Health and Human Services is authorized to put the IPAB recommendations into effect. Savings are likely to come from eliminating excessive payments for robotic surgery or similar exorbitant costs that do not yield better outcomes—not from cutting Granny's pills.

An alternative to the doomsday fear-mongering would be for all Americans to roll up their sleeves and get to work to make the Affordable Care Act the success

our country deserves for it to be. We can also make needed changes in the tax code. We can address the injustice of a shrinking middle class and an ever-increasing poverty class as we repeal the lowest tax rates for the wealthy in more than 70 years. The Ryan/Republican road to prosperity speaks for the rich. The poor absorb 80% of budget cuts in the Ryan plan. The large middle-class loses Medicare after ten years, and the ultra-rich have their taxes lowered from 35% to 25%, while corporate rates are also reduced, giving them larger profits under this Ryan plan. This is indeed "the road to prosperity," but only for the super-rich.

Republican Alternative to the Affordable Care Act

In November of 2010, when Republicans became the majority in the U.S. House of Representatives, they vowed to "repeal and replace" health care reform. On January 19, 2011, the House repealed the Act, as promised, but the action ended in the Senate controlled by the Democrats. The Republicans were less clear about the "replacement" part of their pledge. For their replacement proposal, they trotted out a slightly revised version of the plan they had introduced in 2009, but it has not been brought to a vote. A web site used by House Republicans (www.GOP.gov) stated that their plan, while not yet developed in detail, would include the following principles:

- Expand health savings accounts. The GOP wants to use these tax-sheltered accounts to pay the deductible part of insurance plans that are offered in the private market. As is typical of Republican plans, this proposal would help higher income workers with significant savings accounts and would do nothing to help working families who do not benefit from a tax shelter.

- Allow insurers to operate across state lines. Americans living in states with expensive health insurance (New York) should be able to go to states with cheaper options (Nebraska). Republican lawmakers presented this part of the plan for legislation in early 2011, as the "Health Care Choice Act." Nobody has explained how it could possibly work in practice. Would the insurance company in Nebraska fly patients from New York to Nebraska when they needed less expensive checkups or hospital procedures?

- Medical liability reform. Republicans believe malpractice lawsuits have forced doctors to take out costly insurance policies and to perform unnecessary tests. The GOP wants to prevent "junk lawsuits" and the inefficiencies of "defensive medicine." While this is certainly a legitimate concern, they do not include any proposal that provides fair compensation for persons whose lives are ruined by careless practice or improper treatment.

- Cover patients with pre-existing conditions. Republicans accept the extremely popular part of the ACA that outlaws dropping patients' insurance when they have pre-existing conditions or making their premiums exorbitantly high. They also want to eliminate annual and lifetime spending caps and prevent companies from dropping patients when they get an expensive illness. The GOP would fund this cost by expanding state high-risk pools and reinsurance programs. This keeps high profit clients in the private sector and shifts the burden of high cost clients entirely to government. Their next step is outrage at high government spending and demands for cuts to Medicaid!

- <u>Prohibit taxpayer funding of abortion</u>. The GOP wants a government-wide permanent prohibition on taxpayer funding of abortions. They want a law that goes beyond the so-called Hyde Amendment, which is not a law, but a rider that is attached to funding bills in each appropriation cycle.

When this Republican bill was introduced in 2009, the Congressional Budget Office estimated it would reduce the federal deficit by $68 million over a decade and provide insurance for an additional three million persons. By contrast, the CBO has estimated that the Affordable Care Act will lower the deficit by $210 billion and cover an additional 32 million Americans during that time frame. And CBO does not count any savings from preventive care because it has no credible way to score this, without prior experience.

Funds Blocked for Expanding Medical Training

During the past decade there has been a bi-partisan concern in Congress over the need to bolster the supply of primary care workers—doctors, nurses, physicians assistants and others. The Affordable Care Act recognizes that the shortfall of medical professionals will be even more extensive, given the increased access to health care of 32 million additional persons. The law creates a 15 member National Health Care Workforce Commission to guide the country as it plans for ways to increase the supply to meet the demand. The Commission was named in October of 2010 but it does not have funds to set up an office, employ a staff or meet other basic obligations. President Obama has asked for an appropriation of $3 million for this purpose in the 2012 budget. The Republican House of Representatives has responded by voting to deny the funding, and has further stipulated that the Commission cannot petition Congress for funds. "No new taxpayer dollars will be directed to fund the law," said Conor Sweeney, spokesman for House Budget Committee Chairman Paul Ryan (R. Wis.).

Some 10,000 additional doctors beyond those being trained will be needed over the next five years, beginning in 2014, and the shortage will grow annually, according to the Department of Health and Human Services. The American Medical College projects that by 2025 the shortage of doctors will grow to 130,000 unless we take action. They point out this need is due to increased population, the aging of the U.S. population and the increased access to medical care expected under The ACA.

Apart from this Commission, the ACA includes several strategies to ward off the impending personnel shortages. It expands the National Health Service Corps, the scholarship program for medical students willing to practice in underserved communities. The law sets up Community Health Centers as additional proper sites for resident medical training and expands focus on primary care training. Much of this planning is also on hold until funds become available. Unless Republicans relent or are voted out of office, our only recourse will be to import large numbers of doctors and nurses from other countries, while our own young people lose promising medical careers.   The Republicans have no plausible plan for training needed personnel, only relentless efforts to block the one specified in the Affordable Care Act.

On November 14, 2011, President Obama announced an initiative to provide $1 billion to hire, train and deploy health care workers other than doctors, part of a broader White House agenda to bolster job creation. Grants will go to medical schools, community groups, local governments and others to experiment with different ways to expand the healthcare workforce while reducing the cost of delivering care.   The initiative will seek ways to pass much of the doctors' more routine work to lesser-trained but competent medical providers. The project became part of President Obama's "We Can't Wait" agenda to get the economy moving, despite a Congress that is blocking legislation and appropriations. All projects are expected to be up and running within six months of funding. Health care employment increased by 300,000 during the year before this announcement.   This initiative, with the attendant funding, was built into the Affordable Care Act. It is expected to provide more jobs, while indirectly helping with the shortage of physicians.

Republicans Target Illness Prevention Plans

The Affordable Care Act calls for expanding preventive wellness measures to improve the nation's health and save billions of dollars in medical expenses. The Republican Congress in 2011 has declared its opposition to such measures. They oppose establishing standards for school lunches to make them more nutritious with fewer calories. Republicans do not want government to restrain food companies from marketing sugar and fat products to children. They have especially taken aim at measures to combat obesity among children and adults. They want not only to halt new initiatives but even to roll back initiatives enacted by the previous Congress.

On May 31, 2011, the GOP majority of the House Appropriations Committee approved a House spending plan for 2012 that directed the Department of Agriculture to disband the plan to raise nutritional standards for school breakfasts and lunches. The Committee noted that the meals would cost an extra $7 billion over five years because they would contain fresh fruits and vegetables, whole grain cereals, and low-fat milk. The Committee concluded that the nation could not afford this extravagance when we need to balance the budget. What false economy!

The Bill that passed on November 15, 2011 declared that tomato paste used on pizzas is a vegetable, and thus fulfills the requirement of providing a healthy vegetable each day. This decision results from lobbying efforts of two major pizzas companies, Con Agra and Schwan, who provide a large portion of school food. They make the 4" x 6" school pizza, called by critics, "a veritable chemical concoction made to look like a pizza." What the children are eating is not even a pizza, much less a vegetable. The so-called tomato paste is a concoction of more than a dozen chemicals, including some dried tomato paste.

Nevertheless, this pizza is what kids have grown up with and it is the all-time favorite school lunch food, followed by Tater Tots and fried chicken nuggets. **Republicans are worried that government is going to**

dictate what children eat, while Democrats see that big food companies and their lobbyists are already dictating what they eat--with disastrous results.

The House Appropriations Committee also ordered the Agriculture Department to stop developing guidelines for companies that market food to children. It directed the FDA to exempt grocery and convenience stores and other businesses from the new food labeling regulations, set to take effect in 2012, requiring that calorie information be displayed.

Meanwhile, a panel at the Institute of Medicine designed an easy system for an unsophisticated public to recognize the quality of food products by very simple markings. They proposed labeling based on three ingredients: amount of salt, amount of fat and amount of sugar. If all three ingredients were low enough to be considered "healthy," three stars would be on the package or box. Some packages would not have any stars. Even children could learn to look for three-star items. Shoppers who have clear, simple and prominent labels are most effectively assisted in buying healthy food items. Food companies and their Republican voices in Congress oppose these markings. Walmart, the nation's largest grocer, announced they would work with the law and begin the labeling.

A provision was added by Congressman Denny Rehberg (R. Mont) to block the FDA from issuing rules or guidelines "not based on hard science." While this might sound innocent, it is aimed at blocking the rule that prevents kids from getting hooked on tobacco with the help of Menthol. Menthol masks the harshness of tobacco smoke and appeals to children, while the nicotine does its deadly work of getting them addicted. (Does anyone see the hand of the tobacco lobby?)

Meanwhile the processed food and advertising industries, with Republican support, are lobbying against all required nutrition guidelines, including those on children's food.[41] Their new lobbying organization calls itself the "Sensible Food Policy Coalition." Members include the nation's biggest food companies such as General Mills, Kellogg and PepsiCo, fast food chains and media companies including Viacom and Time Warner, with the U.S. Chamber of Commerce also lending its muscle. This group proposes to issue its own voluntary guidelines to reduce salt, sugar and fat. The U.S. Chamber claims that requiring companies to post nutritional guidelines would kill 75,000 jobs!

Public health experts point out that children, who lack the critical skills to understand advertizing tricks, are subjected to a constant barrage of intriguing cartoons that promote junk food. In a new study of 84 children's cereals from the four big manufacturers,[42] the majority contained more sugar than three chocolate chip cookies. The food and beverage industry spends about $2 billion each year marketing directly to children. The ACA confronts the fact that one in three kids is overweight or obese, a tragic time bomb for future suffering and exploding health care costs. **The American military reports that it can now accept only one in four applicants for enlistment due to obesity, health problems or lack of education.**

The government subsidizes Big Ag—including the biotech and chemical companies that produce pesticides, herbicides, and chemical fertilizers—and Big Food to produce the empty calorie processed foods that are causing so much damage to our nation's health. This is why they are so "cheap" compared with high quality fruits and vegetables. Then Big Pharma reaps untold billions on drugs to treat the resulting diseases. All of these industries have huge government lobbying operations and tight revolving door relationships with the government agencies that are supposed to regulate them. **We cannot abdicate the fate of our nation's health to these entrenched interests.**

To begin to address the devastating public health problems caused by overconsumption of unhealthy processed foods, the Affordable Care Act has charged four government agencies with establishing national nutritional labeling guidelines and determining specific ways that nutritional labeling is to be displayed on all foods that are sold. The guidelines are being finalized and sent back to Congress for final approval. These two powerful forces, the Affordable Care Act and the Republicans in Congress, are moving in opposite directions. They may be at a standstill until one prevails or a compromise is reached.

Republican Presidential Candidates Muddy the Waters

All Republican primary presidential candidates have been in a contest to see who could make the most outlandish claims about how they would destroy the Affordable Care Act. Michele Bachmann and Rick Santorum claimed that on their first day in office they would give immunity to every state to waive all provisions of the law. The problem with this threat is that it cannot be legally carried out. Only partial immunity can be legally granted on an individual provision, and then only with certification that it would be impossible to carry out the provision in reasonable fashion. A time limit must then be provided for rectifying the problem. These two candidates have not read the law.

Rick Perry of Texas railed against the excessive cost of the Act. Then when President Obama proposed a rational way to cut a cost as part of his effort to remove a trillion dollars from the budget over ten years, the Texas Governor denounced the President. Under a 2001 program called "TRICARE for Life" families of military retirees on Medicare receive free additional coverage for their out-of-pocket costs, worth about $2,100 annually. President Obama proposed a modest annual payment reduction in these subsidies, beginning at $200 per person and then rising gradually for a savings of almost $7 billion over ten years. Perry pounced. "Mr. President, the men and women of our military who have served our country with courage every single day have already sacrificed enough." Perry declared, "The least you can do, Mr. President, is to have the courage to cut the government bureaucracy instead of cutting their benefits."

Massachusetts Health Plan after Five Years

In April 2006 Massachusetts became the first state to set the goal of universal coverage for its citizens. In many ways that plan served as a model and guide for the Affordable Care Act, although the new federal program has three goals, rather than one of universal coverage only. Massachusetts created a health insurance exchange, required most citizens to carry insurance, and gave subsidies to those who could not afford the total cost. **As a result, 98% of Massachusetts residents have health insurance at some part of the year and 96% are fully insured on a continuing basis—by far the highest rate in the nation.** The state has a new tax form where people report the kind of health insurance they have.

Fears of government control are proving unfounded. More than 80% of non-elderly residents have private insurance, and 76% of employers offer coverage to their workers, up five percentage points since the program began in 2007. The system that provides insurance for everyone has not resulted in a shortage of doctors, and it is not bankrupting the state even though virtually everyone is covered and costs are rising. Public support for the system remains high.

However, while the state attended to universal coverage, it focused far less on controlling costs and improving quality. "We did access first," said state Senate President Terese Murray (D). "Now, we have to figure out how we can afford it." Governor Deval L. Patrick (D) has riveted his attention on cutting costs without reducing coverage. He is working with the state's insurance companies, medical society, legislature and his own staff to diagnose the problems and offer solutions.

His work has led to a surprising consensus that fee for service medicine is one primary culprit that drives up costs and leads to uneven quality of care. He is proposing a new way to pay for care that follows the new national model of Accountable Care Organizations. The biggest supporter in the state is probably Blue Cross Blue Shield, the Commonwealth's largest health insurer. In 2009, it began a new flat-rate payment system to a group of doctors and hospitals with whom it worked. About a third of the primary care doctors in their network now work for a salary plus incentives, and the number is growing.

Blue Cross Blue Shield has been joined by Partner's Health Care, the Boston-based complex that dominates health care there. Massachusetts General Hospital has launched a Medicare experiment in which nurses coordinate care for 2,500 older patients with multiple illnesses. During the first five years the experiment has reduced medical spending by 7% while hospital re-admissions were lowered by one-fifth. The national plan for dealing with the elderly with multiple illnesses was modeled on this program.

Recently Attorney General Martha Coakley used her subpoena power to get information for a report that showed large disparities in hospital prices. She concluded costs were unrelated to the quality of care, the sickness of patients, or whether it was a teaching hospital. "The only quality that determined cost," she said, "was market leverage." In other words, **hospitals and doctors were charging what they could get away with**.

Meanwhile, the Governor says he has grown impatient with insurance cost increases. The problem has become so urgent that he is ready to step in and determine which increases, if any, the state will permit. Governor Patrick introduced a legislative proposal in February 2011 that would make changes in both private and public insurance plans. He proposed to accelerate the shift to what he terms "global payments" within four years and also give the insurance commissioner authority to reject rate increases proposed by insurance companies. The debate rages over how much control the state should exercise. A large majority believes that changes are proceeding in the right direction. Governor Patrick concludes that there must be accountability by the providers. He said, "I am not persuaded that the market is going to get this right all by itself."[43]

Short-Term Adjustments in the ACA

Republican critics of the law like to say it provides "one size fits all" solutions to local problems of varying kinds. However, a special effort is being made to phase in the law, with deference to local conditions, to create as few local challenges as possible. Two examples will illustrate.

"Mini-Med" health plans, quite common in the past, are being phased out. These low-cost plans provide false assurance to the poor who take them. Some plans pay as low as $2,000 in total life-time benefits, for example. Too many unsuspecting customers think they have insurance only to discover too late that they must fend for themselves when they develop a serious illness. By 2011 mini-meds were mandated to raise their annual coverage limit to $750,000. The plans are supposed to be phased out completely by 2014. Yet more than 2.6 million Americans are still insured under these old plans. Waivers have been granted to 1,040 mini-med plans for 2011 because most of the state insurance exchanges have not yet been set up. Because so many waivers were needed, Republicans charged that the mandates are unattainable. Expectations were based on inaccurate knowledge of the number of people who actually carried that minimal kind of insurance. Before being granted a waiver each company must write to its customers and inform them that their plan fails to meet federal standards, and then direct them to a federal web site where they can search for alternative approved insurance.[44]

Another example of the effort to be flexible is the implementation of the ACA three-year waiver given to Maine regarding the federal mandate that every insurance company must spend at least 80% of its revenue on actual health care. The waiver allows the companies in Maine to continue spending only 60% of premiums on patients, with the rest going toward administration and profits. They were granted a reprieve because the requirement in the short term had "a reasonable likelihood of destabilizing the Maine individual insurance market," wrote Steve Larsen of the Center for Consumer Information and Insurance Oversight. Kentucky, New Hampshire and Nevada have also applied to delay implementation of this rule until exchanges are established, all of them being low population states.

States Prepare to Implement Exchanges

Each state has the complex challenge of setting up its exchange system. This requires enacting legislation and then developing a computer network large enough to include all of the providers, terms of policies, and the capacity to serve all the individuals in the state who are to use the system. This will take time and money. It is supposed be ready for use by January 1, 2014. The Act provides that any state that is not making sufficient progress will have the program placed in the hands of the federal government. No state has the option of defying federal law.

Oklahoma's Republican Governor, Mary Fallin, was thrilled when her state was awarded a health reform innovation grant for which she had applied. Oklahoma was provided $54 million to set up a model computer system that would show the way forward for the rest of the country. Oklahoma had the prospect of free money and an early finish, while being honored for its vision. But, alas, Republican legislators in Oklahoma did not like the idea of cooperating with the Obama Administration. Governor Fallin had to return the money and pretend she hadn't wanted it in the first place.

States across the Midwest and the upper Midwest went heavily Republican in the 2010 election with a split in power between traditional Republicans and new Tea Party activists. Tea Party legislators want nothing to do with setting up exchanges, preferring to wait with the hope that the Supreme Court will rule against the Affordable Care Act or that Republicans will win in the Senate, take back the White House in 2012, and repeal "Obamacare." More circumspect traditional Republicans want to construct their own state exchange programs rather than leave implementation to the federal government.

Minnesota offers an interesting picture of the confusion. The state legislature went Republican but a Democrat, Mark Dalton, captured the Governorship, replacing former Republican Governor Tim Pawlenty. Dalton has been silent on an exchange plan but has generally embraced the Affordable Care Act. State Representative Erin Murphy of the Democratic-Farmer-Labor Party has taken the lead and filed what she terms a "robust" exchange bill. Three-term Republican Steve Glottwald, Chairman of the Health and Human Services

Reform Committee, with 10 years experience in the health care industry, has designed a Republican alternative. However, it has not gained traction among Republicans, especially among new state legislators who proudly wear the Tea Party label. Business groups want exchange legislation enacted to settle the matter and avoid a plan handed down from Washington. Pressure is mounting to enact the state legislation but the Tea Party legislators are resisting.

By December 1, 2011, 29 states had enacted their health insurance exchange legislation. An additional 13 states were awarded $220 million to establish exchanges, including six states led by Republicans who petitioned the Supreme Court to strike down the law. They are Alabama, Arizona, Idaho, Michigan, Maine and Nebraska. The federal government is giving state legislatures until June 29, 2012 to have their exchanges at a specified advanced level of preparation. On that date, they each receive a final grant to complete their exchange, or they will be co-opted by the federal government.

A Related Public Health Issue

The recent focus on America's health has led to fresh consideration of a related issue. The 2011 Senate committee that oversees the Environmental Protection Agency has introduced a bill to address fatal illnesses in children caused by ground toxins in specific localities. The bill drafted by Senators Barbara Boxer (D. Calif.) and Mike Crepo (R. Idaho) is titled, "Disease Clusters and Environmental Health." It is termed "The Trevor Act" in honor of Trevor Schaefer of Idaho, a young man who recently graduated from college after surviving a terrible brain cancer. He has started a Foundation termed the Trevor Trek Foundation to push for and support this type of legislation.

A "disease cluster" is found in a small community where a highly significant number of persons have contracted the same disease, usually some form of cancer. When tracing the problem to its source, the EPA finds that a particular toxic chemical has been dumped into a landfill or stream and has leached into the water supply or the air. Ms. Erin Brockovich, who has dedicated her life to this issue, testified before the Senate Committee that oversees the EPA that she has been called by people in 534 communities around the country who believe they are victims of such chemical dumps. Usually local residents have trouble finding the appropriate government agency to address their concerns, and when they do get through on a telephone call, the person answering is often unresponsive.

The bill, if enacted, will link local communities with experts who will investigate these concerns. It authorizes the EPA to analyze toxins in the bodies of affected individuals and then determine their origin. The goal is to identify the responsible party and require it to pay for cleanup and restitution to aggrieved citizens.

A companion bill is being introduced in the Senate by Frank Lautenburg (D. N.J.) to require testing for every new chemical before it is released into the environment. Is it toxic? For how long is it toxic? One year? One hundred years? **A frightening reality addressed by the Bill is that there are now 80,000 chemicals that have been or are being used today, and only about 200 of them have been**

tested.   New-born babies have hundreds of these environmental toxins in their bodies. Specific chemicals are being linked with specific types of diseases and birth defects.   Yet   most   Republicans   steadfastly   oppose regulation of chemicals.

Considering the enormous increase in the incidence of cancer over the past century, relatively little research has been done on what has caused this horrific devastation. In 1900, about 64 deaths per 100,000 of the population were attributed to some form of cancer. By 2,000, 200.5 persons per 100,000 died of cancer, and this is after billions were spent on research to cure cancer and modern treatments for cancer were put in place.   The unexposed story is that death from cancer has increased remarkably as a vast array of new, untested chemicals flooded our waters, clouded our air, and found their way into the food we eat. Let it be noted that there was a 16% increase in toxic chemicals released into the atmosphere in 2010 alone over the prior year, primarily from a few metal processing industrial sites.

The   American   Chemistry   Council   with   their Republican allies in Congress have urged the EPA to refrain from issuing further regulations or reports to the public.[45] Again, special interests continue to put corporate profits and convenience above public health, prevention of human suffering and the social costs of illness. **Much of the American public seems mesmerized into following meekly while the human causes of cancer fail to rouse our ire. We seem content to spend our money searching for expensive and elusive cures rather than tracking down and removing causes.**

The first of these bills under consideration in the Senate, the Trevor Act, identifies and addresses cancer clusters that now exist. The second seeks to control poisonous chemicals before they are sprayed on our food or otherwise introduced into the environment without regard for public health. Such laws would support the goals of the Affordable Care Act without necessarily becoming part of it. While the bills have some bi-partisan support, they are largely opposed by Republicans in the Senate and find almost no prospect for enactment in the Republican controlled House. Passage must wait for a more humane Congress.

Meanwhile, *Consumer Reports* tested 88 samples of apple and grape juice and found 10% with arsenic levels that exceed federal drinking water standards. They reported that federal standards exist for drinking water but not for bottled juice. Tests show that most of the arsenic and lead found result from human pollution; they are not organic, as found in nature. Only 41% of the samples met standards that *Consumer Reports* considers to be safe.[46] This is but one small example of contamination of our food supply with toxic chemicals. **For genuine health, we *must* have clean food, clean water, and clean air—the basics of life**. Yet the Republican response on how to create jobs and get the economy moving is to get government out of the business of regulating.

Medicare to Enforce Hospital Quality Control

Medicare has been publishing patient satisfaction scores on its Hospital Compare website since 2008. The Center for Medicare and Medicaid Services is finalizing plans to implement a provision of the Affordable Care Act that affects how hospitals are paid. In October 2012, Medicare will begin withholding one percent of its payment to hospitals with poor patient satisfaction and health outcomes. The money goes into a pool, $850 million the first year; it is then distributed to those hospitals that achieve an above average level of satisfaction. The scheme is designed to upgrade the quality of care in all hospitals. Results will be displayed online.

Patients are asked to evaluate their experience. Was the room clean? Were the nurses friendly and responsive? Was pain well controlled? Did the hospital provide instructions for patients to follow when they left the hospital? Patient scores will determine 30 percent of the bonuses, while clinical outcomes and other measures of basic quality will determine the balance.

Television ads, funded by the for-profit hospitals, are flooding the airways showing concerned older persons living in fear that the hospitals will not have funds sufficient to serve them, should they need hospital care.

Costs Continue to Escalate

Before the Affordable Care Act could gain traction with provisions gradually taking effect until 2014, the AARP Price Watch found retail prices for popular brand-name drugs used by seniors increased 8.3% in 2009, while the rate of inflation fell by 0.3%. This appears to be a clear example of price gouging.

The Independent Payment Advisory Board (IPAB), once again was created in the ACA to monitor costs and prevent providers from gouging the system. Republicans oppose the IPAB and claim that it will have too much power. Budget Committee Chairman Paul Ryan (R. Wis.) charged that IPAB will ration needed care for seniors, sending a climate of fear that spread like an out-of-control blaze through the Tea Party.

Senator John D. Rockefeller IV (D. W.Va.), one of the IPAB architects, replied that the Board is prohibited by law from rationing care, restricting benefits or changing eligibility criteria. The purpose of the IPAB is not to restrict older Americans but to set limits on providers who charge outrageous prices to inflate profits. Rockefeller said specifically that **the Board's purpose is to reduce the influence of "special interests" on the Medicare payment policy. These interests, he and others say, have kept Congress from making the tough decisions needed to hold down spending and reduce the deficit.**

Doctors, hospitals, insurance companies, drug companies and medical device makers are all apprehensive. They fear the IPAB will infringe on their ability to raises prices at a rate far higher than the rate of inflation. Under the law, the board is required to recommend reductions in Medicare if spending per capita exceeds preset targets.[47] The Congressional Budget Office projects it will be a full decade before spending begins to spiral out of control. President Obama wants to tighten the IPAB target in later years to GDP plus 0.5% rather than 1% as part of his plan to reduce the deficit. While claiming to be focused on deficit reduction but opposing the cost reduction mandates of the IPAB, Republicans seem intent on preventing cost control.

Looking Ahead

As the country moves into the 2012 election cycle it becomes important to ask what would happen to the Affordable Care Act were Republicans to make electoral gains.

Republican candidates for president vie with each other in claiming to be the most strongly opposed to "Obamacare." They attack the front runner Mitt Romney for having implemented the ACA model in Massachusetts. While we can only speculate on the policy actions any of these candidates might take if elected, it seems reasonable to assume that any of them might go through with his promise to destroy "Obamacare."

Some commentators believe that Romney, once elected, might be more inclined to tweak the law and keep much of it in place, since it is based on his own planning and the law he supported in Massachusetts. His changes might be more incremental. Mr. Romney pledged on the campaign trail to sign an Executive Order his first day in office "to give the states waivers from the law's mandates." The law itself offers that right to states, beginning in 2017, provided they give coverage as strong as what the federal law provides. Romney's policy might, in effect, speed up that right to 2013.

Should Republicans control the House and Senate, they would probably pass a law to repeal the entire Affordable Care Act. Obama would be expected to veto it. But if a Republican were also in the White House a veto would be unlikely.

The drama continues. Final words have not been spoken. The future is ours to shape. Let us turn now to consider a successful way forward.

Chapter 8

CITIZENS UNITE

Reform is not a luxury that can be postponed, but a necessity that cannot wait.
> --President Barak Obama,
> Meeting with health care leaders, May 11, 2009

Gulliver's Travels tells the story of a pygmy race of people who had two political parties. Members of one party wore high-heeled shoes, while members of the other party wore low heels. The low heel party was in power. Although the Crown Prince was thought to favor the high heelers, he wore one heel high and the other one low, causing him to hobble through life. There is a time to settle for compromise, when it supports the common good. But we hobble through life when we choose one high heel and other low. The Affordable Care Act represents a major compromise by most Democrats from a more efficient single payer plan used by virtually all other industrialized countries. This legislation proposed and supported by Republicans in the past offers a bare minimum roadmap of what is necessary in order to substantially meet the three goals of the Act. Further compromise will mean we hobble into an uncertain future.

We have studied the Affordable Care Act and reported on ways the law is being implemented. We have shown how the law is designed to move us to universal coverage, to improve health for everyone, and to carefully manage costs. Success or failure depends in large part, we have insisted, on how well we can learn to view the system as a whole, along with its individual pieces, and then how well that system is managed and improved over time. We have seen the ACA as much a process as a product. It is a way to explore best practices and more sustainable health care options. We are at the beginning, not the end of our great experiment.

Nothing is more important than our health. For good health, as a society, we must focus on support for good health habits, access to healthy food and pure water, and reduction of environmental toxins. This is important both for the wellbeing of our people and for reducing financial pressure on our health care system. From the perspective of the direct concerns of the Affordable Care Act, nothing is more important for millions of us than access to good health insurance. Nothing is more important than the quality of care offered by our doctors and hospitals. And, to have a healthy nation we must control the cost of health care. Yes, even to ensure a healthy economy we must control the cost of health care. In the past, whatever cost saving we have achieved has been through denying coverage. We have now decided that the old approach is no longer appropriate. It is not humane, it is not sustainable, and it is bad business.

The Affordable Care Act represents a huge challenge. It is more a vision of what can be than an accomplishment. In the words of Moses echoed by Martin Luther King Jr., "I have seen the promised land." We have seen what this law offers in prospect, but its fulfillment lies ahead. Cynics abound. They remind us that the powerful special interest groups have billions of dollars at stake. Most of them are not ready to relinquish part of their profits for the sake of the common good. Some jealously guard their wild-west gold mines and will not give up any part of their profits without a last-ditch fight. Strong opponents of the ACA are dedicated to repealing the law or gutting its effectiveness.

The Threat of the Republican Right

A dedicated majority of the Republican Party is bent on repealing this law. Their "repeal and replace" slogan rings hollow. Their "replace" takes us back to the wild-west of health care. The few improvements they propose are like sporadic raindrops trying to fill an ocean of need. Only a determined minority believes that government should not be involved in health care. The majority of Americans who supported passage of the ACA accept a role for free enterprise, but they believe also that health, education and other basic services that promote the general welfare do not lend themselves to a ruthless marketplace dominated by the private profit motive.

The entire field of Republican candidates seeking the 2012 Presidential nomination spoke in virtually every debate with a single voice in their condemnation of the Affordable Care Act. The Florida debate was the one that focused on their larger prescription for the economy. Their answer to every problem—how to create jobs, balance the national budget or deal with the national crisis in health care—was the same litany: cut spending, cut the size of the federal government, cut taxes and protect the wealth of the super rich. They betrayed no empathy for Americans who are desperate to find jobs or obtain health services. Perry,

Governor of Texas, went the extra mile and declared he wants to make the federal government "inconsequential." He thinks Social Security is a "Ponzi scheme" and a "monstrous lie."   He left the strong impression that government workers, including teachers and firefighters, do not have "real" jobs.

The Republican Party realized from the beginning of this debate in 2008 that, if President Obama and the Democratic Party led the effort for a new comprehensive health care system and were able to implement it, the new law would soon gain the same kind of acceptance and support as Social Security and Medicare. Citizens would come to expect health care at a more reasonable price and would fight any effort to take it away. These citizens would put two plus two together and realize it was the Democratic Party that provided this major advance. The Affordable Care Act could solidify Democrats in power for years.

Republicans remember vividly how they defeated the health care law proposed by President and Mrs. Clinton in 1993-1994. They recall how this major defeat led to Republican gains in Congress in the next election. Leaders wanted a repeat performance. South Carolina Republican Senator Jim DeMint summed up his party's view when he said in 2009 that if they are able to stop Obama on health reform, "It will be his Waterloo. It will break him." About that same time Mitch McConnell, the GOP Senate leader, openly discussed his plan to win back the Senate and defeat the President in the 2012 election. It was "absolutely critical" the leader said, that all Republicans stand united to prevent Democrats from passing the health care law and "...be able to say it was bipartisan and thus convey to the public that this law is O.K."

History records that the Republicans did, in fact, stand in solidarity. President Obama spent months trying to find common ground with at least some Republicans, while Senator Max Baucus, Chairman of the Finance Committee, toiled with a "gang of six" — three Republicans and three Democrats — to reach common ground. All was to no avail, except to wear down public expectations and provide time to corrode public support with a concerted chorus of false and misleading claims using hot-button words, such as "death panels," that were carefully tested by Republican operatives.

Republicans at that point no longer looked at the merits of the Act but focused on the politics. They decided to speak with conviction but confuse the public by calling black white. They could, of course, have taken a different tact and cooperated in crafting a law such as the one Republicans led in designing in Massachusetts. They could have had more of an imprint on the final product and gotten as much credit as Democrats for its passage. But that was not to be.

Now Republicans continue to plot strategies for defeating the Affordable Care Act by legislation. They know that if they elect a President in 2012, hold the House and pick up a few more seats in the Senate, they will control all branches of government. Then it will be a rather simple matter to kill the legislation. Seldom has a political election cycle been as important as the one in 2012.

Should they fail to gain control of Congress and the White House, they have two further attack routes. They can get a favorable decision from the U.S. Supreme Court, declaring parts of the law or all of it unconstitutional. If the current court does not strike down the mandate that everyone have insurance before the election, then by gaining a Republican president to replace Barak Obama they would appoint the next Supreme Court judge and tip the scale to an even more conservative court that would outlaw the Affordable Care Act in its present form. With a very conservative majority already in place and with a Republican President who could appoint yet another conservative to the Court, the power would be in their hands to take our nation where they chose.

Another major way to weaken if not destroy the law is by way of the states. The Act wisely gives significant leeway to states so they can craft details of the law to meet their specific needs and preferences, always within basic national guidelines. It becomes hard to hone a vibrant and constructive health care plan when conservative governors and state legislatures dislike the law and are constantly searching for ways to weaken or destroy it.

The Underlying Crisis of Class Warfare

Our nation has now endured as of January 1, 2012 three years of economic crisis. The health care crisis is part of an escalating class war. The gulf is between a Republican party that obediently serves the interests of the very rich and the Democrats who speak for all Americans, while emphasizing justice for the middle class and concern for the poor. The warfare has grown even more intense with the rise of the Tea Party, primarily middle class citizens aligning themselves with the interests of the very wealthy. With the emergence of the Occupy protesters, intending to represent the 99% against the 1% that controls the wealth and most of the power, the conflict is becoming even more polarized.

There is reason for Americans to have the deepest concern. Republican policies since Ronald Reagan have skewed the tax codes and the legislative agendas to favor the rich over the poor and the middle class. Republicans have appointed Supreme Court justices who declare that corporations are individuals, many with incomes in the billions of dollars, who can spend as much on elections as they choose in the name of "free speech." Wealthy individuals and corporate groups have hired a vast army to lobby for their special interests, so often at public expense and against public interests. Is this shift of money and political power real? Is it mere political propaganda? Or are there hard facts to support these claims? Here are some of the salient facts:

- By 2010 the number of Americans without health insurance had ballooned to 49.9 million (U.S. Census Bureau).
- The average annual premium for health insurance for a family of four reached $15,073 in 2011, 9% higher than in 2010—30% of the median family income.
- The number of persons in poverty increased to 46.2 million by 2010, including 22% of the nation's children (U.S. Census Bureau).
- One-third of Americans dropped out of the middle class over the last 30 years (U.S. Census Bureau).

- 18% of Americans said they did not have enough money to buy basic food at times in 2010 (Gallup poll).
- The number of people making more than $5.6 million a year skyrocketed by 385% while the income of the bottom 90% (about 137 million people) remained stagnant during these past 10 years.
- Corporations exploit tax loopholes and favorable tax code provisions to avoid paying taxes altogether, or pay a percentage lower than the average worker. General Electric, for example, generated $10.3 billion in pre-tax income in 2009, paid no U.S. taxes, and actually claimed a tax credit of $1.1 billion.
- Leading candidates for President on the Republican side favor a "flat tax." They describe their plans as ways to simplify the tax code. This sounds good on the surface, but their proposed flat tax would in fact dramatically shift the tax burden even farther onto the middle class, while providing tax savings of millions annually for each corporation and hundreds of thousands for each individual in the upper 1% of incomes.

The Way Forward

The Affordable Care Act disturbs the one percent and their agents in Congress so much because this is the first major social legislation since the Reagan era that reverses the trend of providing more breaks for the rich at the expense of the middle class and the poor. This law is precisely necessary if the goal is once again to embrace the 99%. It is a social contract that looks to the common good.

The years from 2010 to 2014 are designated as the period of time necessary to bring the many parts of the Affordable Care Act into existence and have it woven into the fabric of American life. That does not mean that the health care system is set in stone at the end of that period. It is designed as a work in progress. Indeed, the law envisions constant research and analysis to improve efficiency and learn better methods of health care service.

President Barack Obama must be reelected to ensure the survival of what has been accomplished. Should Democrats also control both the House and Senate, the full measure of the law could become embedded in our society more rapidly. It would then become difficult for any faction to destroy universal health care. It would become almost unthinkable for America to return to its dubious status as the only advanced country in the world without a coherent health care system that provides universal coverage.

One of the persistent threats to the integrity of the law is the ability of the lobbies to influence those in Congress and in state governments. Changes to the policies within the ACA can be made quietly, one small piece at a time. The insurance companies, the hospitals, the doctors, the medical device makers, and the drug companies will all try to win concessions. Some adjustments in their favor may be necessary. However, **an important component in the success of health care in America is to create a public attitude that demands that providers give top priority to the public good.**

Study the successful health care systems in other countries and it becomes apparent that their citizens assume government can and should control costs and offer quality service. Their publics would not tolerate compromises to the integrity of the system or let people be denied care because of low income. The opposite seems to be true in our society. **We somehow assume that it is appropriate for the myriad private providers and corporate players to demand maximum profit without regard for out-of-control costs for consumers or the desperation of the uninsured. That mind-set has to change for us to succeed.**

The long journey from Harry Truman to Barack Obama was an exercise in conviction and determination. Finally, after years of asking Americans to listen to their better angels, Medicare and Medicaid became law. Next in the forward march was the law enacted under Ronald Reagan that forbade hospitals from turning away the nation's uninsured at a time of "life or death" emergency. Then, with one in five of the nation's children without minimum health care, the CHIP program was enacted to cover them. These laws have been incorporated into the Affordable Care Act. Now the even greater challenge is to preserve and expand on the vision expressed in the Affordable Care Act: health care for all, better quality health care for rich and poor alike, and control of costs that threaten to bankrupt us. Let's keep moving forward! Let's keep believing in ourselves as a nation where our "better angels" prevail!

Those of us who support the vision of universal coverage, quality health care for everyone, and controlled costs do not need to wait passively for election returns in our favor. We can form citizens' organizations to support our demands and influence our law makers. We will need a citizens' lobby along the lines of the American Association of Retired Persons (AARP). We will also need one or more policy research foundations along the lines of the conservative Heritage Foundation to study specific issues, make recommendations, and serve as a "watch-dog" over the system. For how long will we need to be on guard? **Eternal vigilance is the price to pay for meaningful health care reform.**

The Larger Crisis: Finding a Common Vision

The greater crisis among us is the crisis of finding a common vision that binds our nation and rallies our citizens. The new vision embraces the common good that reaches beyond private interests, transcends sectarian favoritism and offers a way to save the earth from destruction by human greed. We face a crisis because one of the dominant narratives of our nation resists the common good and denies a common destiny.

The familiar narrative of favoritism is framed like this: America is the land of freedom, including freedom to invest, invent and prosper. Government is the enemy, because when we turn our freedom over to bureaucrats they make stupid rules that impede the freedom of the market. Government stifles business and rewards poor performance with grants and subsidies to the under-achievers. We must return to the era of small government and unshackle the hands of the masters of industry who provide jobs. We must lower taxes on those who design new businesses so we can all prosper. In the end, all of our social ills, including the need for job creation, can be traced to over-regulation and high taxes, especially on large corporations and the top one percent. Rolling back the

Affordable Care Act is an important part of getting government off our backs.

A surprising number of distressed and discouraged people in the lower economic brackets buy into this narrative and accept its premise. Government appears to be failing to provide jobs and security. In their search for a reasoned explanation, they find "answers" from Murdock-controlled media and a political party that views government as the enemy. They like lowering taxes, even when their own rates are already relatively low. Those who create this narrative know it represents the interests of only a small minority when it is presented alone, so they enlist the support of the religious right who believe the ills of society can be traced to such things as homosexuality, birth control and abortion. By cleverly weaving that narrative into their economic agenda, the alternative vision gains the support of a significant percentage of the population. By tacitly accepting a pre-scientific interpretation of scripture and a vision of America as a "Christian" nation, according to the religious right's narrow interpretation of Christianity, the one percent has a plan for domination.

The grand vision toward which we move sees our nation on a journey toward the common good. We appreciate and find solace in our family histories, our ethnicity, our race, our sect, and our political party. We embrace the good they provide for us. Nonetheless, we refuse to worship at any of their shrines because our vision lies beyond their limited scope. We are inclusive. We want all citizens to be afforded rights. We will not stop until the rich, by consent or by force of law, pay their fair share and join the search for the common good. We will camp on the doorstep of Wall Street until there are necessary regulations to protect that common good and until those who choose to circumvent the law are brought to justice.

The case for the common good is presented as an epic struggle between the 1% and 99%, or between the self-centered powerful against those who pursue the general welfare. However, in the real world the division between "good" and "evil," or "us vs. them" is never this clear. There are very wealthy people with generous spirits who care deeply, contribute generously, and work tirelessly for the common good. There are people at every income level who are selfish and narrow minded. We note that most of those who work for the wellbeing of others and support civic health through gladly paying taxes are happier than those working to push others aside for their individual advantage alone. While acknowledging these nuances, **we still discern a "dominant narrative" that seeks control of the political and economic arenas for narrow and destructive ends.**

We affirm that the many thousands of people who work in health-related fields and are part of organizations that seek special advantage are not evil people. They perceive themselves as servants of the common good who nonetheless want to protect and enhance their own stake in the system.

Our grand vision is of a nation that demands that elected representatives work for the larger public, not for special interests that bleed the national treasury to increase their own profits. It is a land that insists that elections be funded by the public, so that those who serve can do the people's business, rather than spend their time raising money for the next campaign.

This society toward which we aspire does not forget the weak, the sick and the dying. It works for release of millions of poor youth in prisons, using the public funds that pay for incarceration for rehabilitation and renewal. It is a people who take seriously the scientific evidence that earth itself is in the deepest of trouble. It is a land where the air is pure and the water clean. We seek a nation where no child goes to bed hungry; indeed, where public policy makes poverty obsolete.

Our grand vision is one in which corporations recognize duty and loyalty to our common good. They no longer use nations as pawns in their game to maximize global profit and power. They are asked to serve the common good of both their nation and the larger world community. They see their purpose as far greater than profit for shareholders and huge pay checks for executives. No longer do companies feel free to blithely move from the communities that have invested in them. They are partners on a common journey with their employees because each paid worker is a person who deserves a measure of security and a share of profits, the fruits of their labor.

Our grand vision will trump their limited, selfish, and pre-scientific vision. **In the end, the struggle is about which vision of a new world we want to create.** It is a classic, profound struggle between their money and our determination. It is a contest between the fear they generate and the hope we proclaim. We will prevail!

ACKNOWLEDGEMENTS

Life has gifted me with far more than I could ever contribute in the area of health care policy. I do want to acknowledge with appreciation persons who volunteered to contribute to the expertise and professionalism of this book.

Elizabeth Bass, Ph.D. is a health economist. She read selected chapters and gave valued insight, especially in the area of cost control. While she is far more cautious than I about the amount of cost savings that can be expected, I value her counsel and appreciate being made aware of factors to be considered that I might have overlooked without her help.

Tom Harter spent a career as a benefits consultant, designing health care plans for Fortune 500 companies and for major labor unions. He showed me how much of the ACA is based on pioneering work in cost control by large business and labor. He detailed for me how major corporations design their own health care plans and self-insure them. He offered both perspective and specific insight.

John DuMoulin holds a key position with the Blue Cross Blue Shield Association. He read several chapters, offered insightful comments and cleared up some potential inaccuracies.

Dana L. Whitley, IOM, is a health care policy analyst who focuses her work on state health policy and legislation. She works for a non-profit professional association that tracks health care policy decisions at both the federal and state levels. She is knowledgeable on the issues and added her insights. In addition, she edited early drafts of several chapters.

Each of these friends is a fellow member of The Falls Church Episcopal where my wife Peggy and I worship and serve regularly.

My greatest debt of gratitude is reserved for Susanna MacGregor, my daughter. In the Prologue Memoir she was the five year old Suzy who had her tonsils taken out under the new health care system in Scotland. Now she is the editor who has worked with patience and perseverance to help shape my drafts into a coherent book. She also contributed valuable insight on the issues.

My son David McCan and his wife Cindy read parts of the final manuscript and offered further suggestions. David, a computer professional, volunteered to set up and support my website and blog for a continuing discussion on the Affordable Care Act and the issues surrounding it.

Jason Fleming, my stepson, is an accomplished graphic design specialist. He designed the cover with the kind of image I sought and did it with artistic excellence.

Finally, I thank Peggy, my wife, for her support of the project and for sharing this driving dream with me. Among her many contributions is her dedicated work as a manager at a large full-service senior living facility.

END NOTES

Prologue: A Medicare Memoir

[1] Ten years after enrolling as a Visiting Scholar at Harvard University with the intention of starting an experimental international college, the vision was realized in embryonic form. Dag Hammarskjold College was established in Columbia, Maryland. It was a bold experiment, underfunded, and many said a couple of generations ahead of its time. It was based on the concept that many years later took root in the cultural mind as "multicultural" education. We had students, faculty and board members from all over the world. We were the only college ever to have internships at the United Nations. Norman Cousins, owner/editor of *The Saturday Review*, served as Chairman of the Board. In the end, my greatest disappointment in life came when we closed for insufficient funds to properly succeed. I still receive emails from former students scattered across the globe who say their international vocations were molded by their experiences at the college.

[2] *Congressional Record*, 7 April 1965.

Chapter 1—The Affordable Care Act: An Overview

[3] The Government Printing Office provides the full text of the Act online: http://purl.access.gpo.gov/GPO/LPS124425.

[4] Richard Nixon, Special Message to the Congress Proposing a Comprehensive Health Insurance Plan,

February 6, 1974. For full text, see: http://www.presidency.ucsb.edu.

[5] Cohen, R.A., Martinez, M.E. "Health Insurance Coverage: Early Release of Estimates From the National Health Interview Survey, January–March 2011." Division of Health Interview Statistics, National Center for Health Statistics, Center for Disease Control and Prevention, September 2011.

[6] "ObamaCare and Carey's Heart." Op-ed by Ron Johnson in *TheWall Street Journal*, March 23, 2011.

[7] Baicker, Katherine, Cutler, David, Song, Zirui. "Workplace Wellness Programs Can Generate Savings." *Health Affairs*, (February 2010): 304-311.

Chapter 3 — Quality Health Care

[8] Boodman, Sandra. "Effort to End Surgeries On Wrong Patient Or Body Part Falters." *Kaiser Health News*, 20 June 2011.

[9] Longman, Phillip. "Best Care Anywhere." *Washington Monthly*, January/February 2005.,

[10] Klein, Ezra. "The Health of Nations." *The American Prospect*, 22 April 2007.

[11] "Shocking news: Overdoing ICDs." *Harvard Health Letter*, March 2011, Vol. 36, No. 5.

[12] Bass, Carole. "The Heart of the Matter." *Yale Alumni Magazine*, July/August, 2011.

[13] Kulkarni, Sandeep C., Levin-Recor, Alison, Ezzati, Majid, Murray, Christopher J.L. "Falling behind: life expectancy

in US counties from 2000 to 2007 in an international context." *Population Health Metrics* 2011, 9:16 (15 June 2011).

Chapter 4—Cost Control

[14] "A wild card in health-care law's new deal." *The Washington Post,* 7 August 2011, G3.

[15] "Medicare fraud crackdown nabs 91 in 8 cities across U.S." *The Washington Post,* 8 Sept. 2011, A3.

[16] "Many hospitals overuse double CT scans, driving up costs, data show." *The Washington Post,* 19 June 2011, A5.

[17] "An expensive radiation therapy focuses attention on centers owned by the physicians who help fill them with patients. Are 'self-referrals' PROPER?" *The Washington Post,* 1 March 2011, E1.

[18] "Is robotic surgery better?" *Harvard Health Letter,* May 2011, Vol. 36, No. 7.

[19] "Private Medicare prices to decrease." *The Washington Post,* 16 September 2011, A10.

[20] "Pricey drugs may not be better." *The Washington Post,* 16 January 2012, E3.

[21] Letter dated August 7, 2009 from Douglas Elmendorf, Director, Congressional Budget Office to Hon. Nathan Deal, Ranking Member, Subcommittee on Health, Committee on Energy and Commerce, U.S. House of Representatives.

[22] Flegal K.M., Graubard B.I., Williamson D.F., et al. "Cause-Specific Excess Deaths Associated With Underweight, Overweight, and Obesity." *Journal of the American Medical Association.* 2007; 298(17):2028–2037.

[23] Anderson D.R., Whitmer R.W., Goetzel R.Z., et al. "The relationship between modifiable health risks and group-level health care expenditures." *American Journal of Health Promotion.* 2000;15:45–52.

[24] Orme-Johnson DW, Walton K. "All approaches to preventing and reversing effects of stress are not the same." *American Journal of Health Promotion.* 1998;12: 297-299.

[25] www.tm.org/research-on-meditation.

[26] www.heartmath.org/research/research-library/research-library.html.

[27] Herron, Robert E., Ph.D. "Changes in Physician Costs Among High-Cost Transcendental Meditation Practitioners Compared With High-Cost Nonpractitioners Over 5 Years." *American Journal of Health Promotion,* September/October 2011, Vol. 26, No. 1, pp. 56-60.

[28] Cohen S.B., Rohde F. "The Concentration in Health Expenditures over a Two Year Time Interval, Estimates for the US Population, 2005–2006." Washington, DC: Agency for Healthcare Research and Quality; April 2009.

[29] Stanton M.W., Rutherford M.K. "The High Concentration of US Health Care Expenditures."

Rockville, Md: Agency for Healthcare Research and Quality; 2005.

[1] Berk M.L., Monheit A.C. "The concentration of health care expenditures, revisited." *Health Affairs*. 2001;20:9-18.

[1] "High-Cost Medicare Beneficiaries." Washington, DC: Congressional Budget Office, Congress of the United States; 2005.

[1] Thorpe KE, Howard DH. "The rise in spending among Medicare beneficiaries: the role of chronic disease prevalence and changes in treatment intensity." *Health Affairs*. 2006;25:w378–w388.

[1] Kurtz, Stanley. "IPAB, Obama, and Socialism." *National Review Online*, 18 April 2011.

[1] "Affordable Care Act Update: Implementing Medicare Cost Savings." Office of the Actuary, Center for Medicare and Medicaid Services, 2010.

Chapter 5 — Health Care in Other Countries

[1] Yglesias, Matthew. "Health Care in Sweden." *Think Progress*, 1 October 2009

Chapter 6 — Moral Issues

[1] Chaves, Mark and Wineburg, Bob. "Did the Faith-Based Initiative Change Congregations?" *Nonprofit and Voluntary Sector Quarterly*, April 2010; Vol. 39, pp 343-355.

[1] Wilper, A.P., Woolhandler, S., Himmelstein, D.U. et al. "Health Insurance and Mortality in US Adults." *American Journal of Public Health*, Vol. 99, No. 12, (December 2009) pp. 2289-2295.

[1] "Graduation lessons." *The Washington Post*, 14 May 2011, A19.

[1] "Economic Justice for All: Pastoral Letter on Catholic Social Teaching and the U.S. Economy." United States Conference of Catholic Bishops, August 2011.

[1] 1 John:3:17.

Chapter 7—Republican Response

[1] "Food, ad industries lobby against nutrition guidelines." *The Washington Post*, 10 July 2011, A3.

[1] "Kids' Cereals Pack More Sugar Than Twinkies and Cookies." Environmental Working Group News Release, 7 December 2011.

[1] "Mass. may revamp health-care payments." *The Washington Post*, 16 April 2011, A2.

[1] "Controversial 'mini-med' plans get reprieves through waivers." *The Washington Post*, 28 March 2011, A15.

[1] "EPA: Toxic chemicals released up 16% in 2010." *The Washington Post*, 6 January 2012, A11.

[1] "Arsenic in your juice: How much is too much? Federal limits don't exist." *Consumer Reports*, January 2012.

[1] "Debate over a new board's role in containing Medicare cost spiral." *The Washington Post*, 8 May 2011, A15.

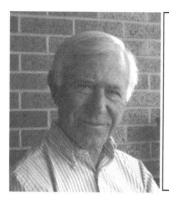

ABOUT THE AUTHOR

Robert L. McCan is a graduate of Yale University Divinity School. He received his Ph.D. from the University of Edinburg, Scotland and continued his education as a Visiting Scholar with faculty status at Harvard University.

Dr. McCan is an ordained Southern Baptist minister and began his career holding pastorates in three churches with 600 to 1,800 members. Dr. McCan founded and served as President of Dag Hammarskjold College. With a majority of students, faculty and Board from other countries, the international college created a miniature world community on campus.

His career in government included executive positions in four federal agencies: the Office of Economic Opportunity; U.S. Office of Education; Woodrow Wilson International Center for Scholars; and the U.S. Agency for International Development.

Dr. McCan also taught and consulted in the field of public policy. He was Assistant Professor of Political Ethics at Wesley Theological Seminary and an Associate at the Churches Center for Theology and Public Policy, sponsored by mainline Protestants and the Roman Catholic Church to assist in developing positions on public policy.

Dr. McCan's previous books include *A Vision of Victory*, *World Economy and World Hunger*, and *Justice for Gays and Lesbians: Crisis and Challenge in the Episcopal Church*. He is married to Peggy McCan. They live in Falls Church, Virginia and are members of Falls Church Episcopal, where he serves on the Vestry.

Made in the USA
Charleston, SC
01 September 2013